Professional Chaplaincy: What Is Happening to It During Health Care Reform?

Professional Chaplaincy: What Is Happening to It During Health Care Reform? has been co-published simultaneously as *Journal of Health Care Chaplaincy,* Volume 10, Number 1 2000.

Professional Chaplaincy: What Is Happening to It During Health Care Reform?

Larry VandeCreek, DMin
Editor

Professional Chaplaincy: What Is Happening to It During Health Care Reform? has been co-published simultaneously as *Journal of Health Care Chaplaincy*, Volume 10, Number 1 2000.

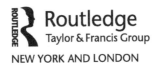

Routledge
Taylor & Francis Group

NEW YORK AND LONDON

First published in 2000 by The Haworth Press, Inc.
10 Alice Street, Binghamton, NY 13904-1580

Published 2017 by Routledge
711 Third Avenue, New York, NY 10017, USA
2 Park Square, Milton Park, Abingdon, Oxon OX14 4RN

Routledge is an imprint of the Taylor & Francis Group, an informa business

Professional Chaplaincy: What Is Happening to It During Health Care Reform? has been co-published simultaneously as *Journal of Health Care Chaplaincy*™, Volume 10, Number 1 2000.

The development, preparation, and publication of this work has been undertaken with great care. However, the publisher, employees, editors, and agents of The Haworth Press and all imprints of The Haworth Press, Inc., including The Haworth Medical Press® and Pharmaceutical Products Press®, are not responsible for any errors contained herein or for consequences that may ensue from use of materials or information contained in this work. Opinions expressed by the author(s) are not necessarily those of The Haworth Press, Inc.

Cover design by Thomas J. Mayshock Jr.

Library of Congress Cataloging-in-Publication Data

Professional chaplaincy : what is happening to it during health care reform? / Larry VandeCreek, editor.
    p . cm.
    Includes bibliographical references and index.
    ISBN 0-7890-1172-7 (alk. paper) – ISBN 0-7890-1173-5 (alk. paper)
    1. Chaplains, Hospital. 2. Health care reform I. VandeCreek, Larry.
BV4335 .P76 2000
259'.4–dc21

00-039661

ISBN 13: 978-0-7890-1173-2 (pbk)

Professional Chaplaincy: What Is Happening to It During Health Care Reform?

CONTENTS

ABOUT THE EDITOR

Larry VandeCreek, DMin, BCC, is Director of Pastoral Research at The HealthCare Chaplaincy in New York City. For the past 23 years, he held faculty and staff positions with The Ohio State University College of Medicine and Public Health and its associated medical center. Dr. VandeCreek is a member of numerous professional associations including the American Association of Marriage and Family Counselors, the Association of Professional Chaplains, Inc., the American Association of Pastoral Counselors, and the Association for Clinical and Pastoral Education. He has published many journal articles which examine aspects of the relationship between religious faith and illness. Dr. Vande-Creek is the author of *A Research Primer for Pastoral Care and Counseling* (Journal of Pastoral Care Publications, 1988) and is Co-Editor of *The Chaplain-Physician Relationship* (1991). He is Editor of the *Journal of Health Care Chaplaincy* (The Haworth Press, Inc.) which has published *Ministry of Hospital Chaplains: Patient Satisfaction* (1997), *Scientific and Pastoral Perspectives on Intercessory Prayer: An Exchange Between Larry Dossey, M.D. and Health Care Chaplains* (1998), *Spiritual Care for Persons with Dementia: Fundamentals for Pastoral Practice* (1999), and *Contract Pastoral Care and Education: The Trend of the Future?* (1999).

Preface

In an article titled "Remembering the Real Questions," J. J. Cohen (1998) wrote that patients primarily ask physicians three central questions: "What is happening to me?" "What's going to happen to me?" and "What can be done to improve what happens to me?" It appears that health care professionals are asking those questions of themselves as reform efforts roll over them. These professions are changing forever. Fox (1998), in fact, suggests that this is the third reorganization of health care, the first beginning in the 1880s as physicians began to use "laboratory science as the basis of useful knowledge about the causes, natural history, and treatment of disease" (p. 314). The second began during the Second World War and continued until recently during which health policy gave priority to supplying as many physicians, particularly specialists, as possible. The third is the reforming process as we know it today.

Professional chaplains are asking these questions too. What is happening to us? What's going to happen to us? What can be done to improve what happens to us? Health care reform is having its own impact on the profession. Increased scrutiny is everywhere and more productivity is expected of everyone. Some departments are losing professional and support positions as well as other resources. The pastoral care profession as we have known it during this century is changing forever.

The professional chaplaincy profession is vulnerable in unique ways when compared to the rest of health care, however. These vulnerabilities have existed for decades, but the reform efforts make them particularly evident and painful. For example, professional chaplaincy

[Haworth co-indexing entry note]: "Preface." VandeCreek, Larry. Co-published simultaneously in *Journal of Health Care Chaplaincy* (The Haworth Pastoral Press, an imprint of The Haworth Press, Inc.) Vol. 10, No. 1, 2000, pp. xi-xv; and: *Professional Chaplaincy: What Is Happening to It During Health Care Reform?* (ed: Larry VandeCreek) The Haworth Pastoral Press, an imprint of The Haworth Press, Inc., 2000, pp. xi-xv. Single or multiple copies of this article are available for a fee from The Haworth Document Delivery Service [1-800-342-9678, 9:00 a.m. - 5:00 p.m. (EST). E-mail address: getinfo@haworthpressinc.com].

lacks national statistical descriptions of itself and how managed care efforts are effecting it. That is, professions such as medicine, nursing, and those in the allied health field all possess studies that provide baseline information concerning the size, shape, and character of their professions. This is also true of psychology, social work, as well as marriage and family therapy. They can quickly provide information concerning the basic characteristics of their professions and answer the question, "Who are we?"

For these professions, such information constitutes the foundation for addressing the question, "What is happening to us?" Given their baseline of information, physicians and hospitals can examine the effects of health care reform on the number of admitted patients and, in fact, provide those details according to hospital size and geographic location. The nursing profession can report the impact of health care reform on the nurse-patient ratio in hospitals, the effects on salary schedules, and changes in the number of overtime hours. Such information contributes to a clearer sense of "what can be done to improve what happens . . . " in the future.

And in the field of professional chaplaincy? Well, little information of this nature exists. The other day a chaplain phoned this editor and asked, "How many chaplains are there in the US?" No one knows! "How many faith-based health care institutions have chaplains?" We don't know? "How many one-chaplain pastoral care departments exist?" We don't know! We don't know the answers to these and a thousand other relevant questions. Thus it has been practically impossible to know in concrete detail what is happening to professional chaplaincy during health care reform. This work seeks to answer some of those questions.

What accounts for this amazing lack of information? One simple reason is that professional chaplains, in contrast to other health care professionals, are not licensed by the state. State licensure boards are often the central registries of such information and professional chaplaincy lacks this centralization. The Coalition on Ministry in Specialized Settings (COMISS) has attempted to create a broad, non-intrusive umbrella, but its various member organizations have not granted it sufficient power so as to generate many obvious benefits.

This is not the only reason for the lack of knowledge, however. It seems that professional chaplaincy is not interested in or does not see the merit of such self-knowledge. For example, after some urging a few years ago, the Association for Clinical Pastoral Education (ACPE) appointed a "Down-Sizing Committee" in 1996 to study what was happening in its education centers. This seemed wholly appropriate given the advance of health care reform. Some hoped that the Committee would create concrete information about the pastoral care and education profession and the impact of reform. The Committee met only a few times before the ACPE Board of representatives dissolved it in 1997.

Another reason is also important. Unlike most other health care professions, professional chaplaincy has no academic arm, no programs (or very, very few) that grant graduate degrees in the field. Thus there are few faculty members and graduate students, few dissertations, and few professional careers built on producing research in the field. All other health care professions have academic programs that anchor, train, and research their clinical activities. One cannot argue that seminaries and their faculties fill this role for institutional chaplaincy; they simply have not done so and for good reasons. Seminaries and their faculties either train persons for a wide variety of graduate studies or provide education for parish ministry. Graduate studies in professional chaplaincy are simply beyond the scope of their mission and curricula. This is a systemic problem and it will not go away any time soon. This lack of academic grounding for the profession will continue to influence the way chaplains think and practice. How different it would be if even 20 tenure-eligible faculty were teaching and publishing their research in the field of professional chaplaincy.

Knowledge creates power, in this instance the power to respond to health care changes in creative ways. Abraham Lincoln had it right when he said that if we could first know where we are and whither we are tending, we could then better judge what to do and how to do it. This publication is offered in that spirit and as a small, beginning effort to answer those three questions that chaplains are asking.

The first piece is a chaplain's story about losing his position due to health care reform. It reflects the individual, human aspects of reform efforts. This is followed by attention to its impact on the profession in the broadest terms. It consists of a report concerning responses from 370 pastoral care department directors to a questionnaire study. In very concrete terms, it answers the question, "What is happening to us?" I think you will find the answers somewhat surprising. Additionally, the department directors rank strategies they have used and will use in the future to deal with downsizing threats.

The third article reports analysis results from the last item in this questionnaire that invited respondents to write narratives concerning their experiences with and concerns about health care reform. Dr. Patrice McCarthy, a nurse with training in the analysis of narrative content, read these narratives and provides a summary of their contents. Again, the results produce an interesting perspective on "What is happening. . . ."

The fourth contribution is an Australian study demonstrating that health care reform is not just a U.S. problem. Even more importantly, however, it names the philosophic foundations of current reform efforts as well as reports some research results concerning chaplaincy on that continent.

The fifth piece again describes the experience of a chaplain, one who is a department manager. The opening story along with this second experience provides brackets for the more impersonal research results. But there is more to the importance of this last story than is immediately apparent. The research results reported above demonstrate that a substantial number of pastoral care departments have actually grown during reform. What could explain that? Certainly it is not the attention to costs! Increasing the number of chaplains in a department costs money! The results suggest a hidden variable, something else that is influencing administrative decisions in such instances. What could it be? In a case study format, this author describes his particular institution and its department. The moral of this story is, "It's not just the cost, stupid; it's also the values embodied by the administration." In unmistakable terms, he links the values held by the CEO to the funding of the pastoral care department. Both the coming and going of this CEO is directly linked to how the department expanded and now is contracting. Presumably, if a new administrator holds values compatible with the ministry of professional chaplaincy the Department will stabilize once again.

Frank Moyer draws attention to interesting materials that provide some unique perspectives on what is happening to the profession and what we can do about it. Noel Brown, editor of The Orere Source, provides both commentary and citations to relevant literature. We owe all of these contributors our thanks.

To the curious and inquisitive reader, the materials in this work may raise as many questions as they answer. That is success; knowing the questions is the first step to finding answers. Even the present results, however, will help the profession begin to make a response to those three primary questions: What is happening to us? What is going to happen to us? and What can be done to improve what happens?

With appreciation, financial support for the questionnaire study is acknowledged from the ACPE Endowment Fund and the ACPE East Central Region.

Larry VandeCreek, DMin, BCC

REFERENCES

Cohen J.J. 1998. Remembering the real questions. *Annual of Internal Medicine*, 128(7), 563-566.

Fox D.M. 1998. Managed care: The third reorganization of health care. *Journal of the American Geriatric Society*, 46(3), 314-317.

CONTRIBUTIONS

My Experience with Health Care Reform

Charles B. Terrell, MDiv

SUMMARY. Health care reform efforts have personal and professional implications as well as consequences. This case study describes the author's experience with suddenly losing his chaplaincy position because of budgetary constraints. Methods of coping with the trauma are described. *[Article copies available for a fee from The Haworth Document Delivery Service: 1-800-342-9678. E-mail address: <getinfo@haworthpressinc.com> Website: <http://www.haworthpressinc.com>]*

KEYWORDS. Clergy, chaplain, pastoral counseling, pastoral care, health care reform

For me personally, health care reform began at three p.m. on December 7, 1998. That is when my pager sounded, asking me to call the Pastoral Care Department. When I returned the page, the Director said that something had come up and that he needed me to come to his

Address correspondence to: Charles B. Terrell, 224 High Street, Berea, OH 44017-1835.

[Haworth co-indexing entry note]: "My Experience with Health Care Reform." Terrell, Charles B. Co-published simultaneously in *Journal of Health Care Chaplaincy* (The Haworth Pastoral Press, an imprint of The Haworth Press, Inc.) Vol. 10, No. 1, 2000, pp. 1-6; and: *Professional Chaplaincy: What Is Happening to It During Health Care Reform?* (ed: Larry VandeCreek) The Haworth Pastoral Press, an imprint of The Haworth Press, Inc., 2000, pp. 1-6. Single or multiple copies of this article are available for a fee from The Haworth Document Delivery Service [1-800-342-9678, 9:00 a.m. - 5:00 p.m. (EST). E-mail address: getinfo@haworthpressinc.com].

office. I was providing follow-up support from a weekend on call to a family with a loved one in the Intensive Care Unit. The patient's condition was deteriorating and the family was struggling through a decision about terminally weaning her from ventilator support. I asked if it could wait until the family had reached a decision and he replied that I needed to come immediately. I was puzzled; this was unusual. I asked if he could give me some idea as to what this was about and he replied that it was not something he wanted to discuss on the phone. I left the family, saying that I had been called away and that I would return as soon as possible.

Arriving at the Director's office, I found him sitting with the Administrator who oversees pastoral care and I began to wonder if there was a problem with some other on-call occasions I had during the weekend. To my complete surprise, the Administrator told me that two staff chaplain positions, including mine, were being eliminated immediately. My colleague and I were permanently laid-off. We could leave now or chose to work through December 31; regardless of our choice, they would pay us through the end of the year.

For the next hour, I experienced almost all of the so-called "stages of grief" compressed into a swirl of surreal emotions. I was shocked; I was in denial; I bargained; I felt depressed; I felt angry; I felt nothing; I felt afraid, I felt so alone. I did not, however, achieve acceptance.

Neither the Administrator nor the Director could adequately explain the rationale for the decision. The Administrator stated that the organization's projected deficit was so bad that cuts had to be made somewhere. One nurse case manager was also laid-off. No one else in this Administrator's area was affected by the cost reductions.

I left the department offices at four p.m. and went, in a daze, to my office. I paged my colleague who had been informed a few minutes earlier than me and she came to my office where we did a mini-debriefing, attempting to support and encourage each other as much as we could. Our family situations are different–I am nearly 49, married with two college-age children; she is sixty, widowed, and anticipates retiring in two years. Nonetheless, the pain and hurt were equally severe. How could this be? Pastoral care was well integrated throughout the hospital; she covered the ICU, the Ortho-Neuro Unit, the Oncology Unit, and the Transitional Care Unit. My areas included the Behavioral Health Unit, the Coronary Care Unit, the Cardiac Step-Down Unit, and Cardiac Rehab Stress Management Education, and

Surgical areas. With the Director, we shared in overnight and weekend on-call rotations and in supervising 35 Stephen Ministers who gave spiritual care to patients referred to us by Home Health and the Outpatient Social Workers. Five Stephen Ministers also provided weekly visitation on the in-patient areas. Another Stephen Minister coordinated the two on-going Bereavement Support groups for the community. Neither she nor I could fully grasp that our participation in all these healing ministries was ended.

At five p.m. I drove to the nearby bus stop to pick up my wife who was coming home from her work. After numerous deep breaths and countless repetitions of The Serenity Prayer, I collected myself and told her what had happened. Her responses mirrored many of my earlier feelings and yet as we sat in the car for several minutes, she was able to speak powerful words that have kept us going; "We'll be okay; we'll make it." Such hope . . . confidence . . . trust. I was unable to generate such confidence myself; she was able to begin to nudge our focus forward to "What do we do next?"

The next day I came to work and became so powerfully aware of the blessings of being connected to the Association of Professional Chaplains and its caring leadership. The notion of being told that I could work (or not) until the end of the year and receive pay regardless of my choice felt and sounded like immediate termination without notice. I called the Association's national office seeking advice and was helpfully given the direct office number of the President.

I dialed and he answered. After empathizing and supporting me upon hearing my story, he helped me to realize that there is a legal business tactic called "giving pay in lieu of notice," and that's what I had received. Beyond that help in understanding, I received valuable grace and encouragement from him during our talk. He told me that he would post my name in the national office and would communicate my need to the Board of Directors by e-mail. I received caring ministry in a time of great fear and uncertainty. Later that week, I received a moving letter and prayer from the Organization's president-elect; several weeks later I received a call from another Board Member, telling me about an available position. He said the Board had been praying for us.

Over the next two weeks my colleague and I went about the painful process of letting the nurses and other staff members know of the decision. The outpouring of their feelings was overwhelming. People were shocked, disbelieving, angry at the Administration, seeking ways to thank us for our eight years of effective and meaningful ministry to and with them, their patients, and to families. My colleague's last day was December 18th; mine was the 23rd. Through these closure efforts, I continued to experience a wide range of emotions. I was aware of the sincere gratitude I felt for being able to work with such tremendous people. At the same time, I also felt anger and resentment toward the Administration for discarding my vital ministry. The staff realized, as did we, that eliminating our two positions would drastically weaken the clinical services provided to patients and families. The staff had always counted on us to be there, even through the most horrible situations. Reducing the Pastoral Care team by two-thirds contradicted the Mission Statement of the hospital that pledged sincere attention to the spiritual needs of patients and families.

In our eight years, my colleague and I made meaningful contributions to hundreds of persons who were in spiritual distress. We frequently intervened to rescue the organization from potentially litigious situations through our ministry to angry patients and families. Our value to the organization could also be measured by the countless acts of good will and positive public relations that we provided to the community at large. Indeed, the groundswell of protest that the hospital received from area churches and numerous volunteers bears this out. Letters to the Editor appeared in the local newspaper; several of the Stephen Ministers wrote to Administration and voiced their displeasure. Many Alcoholics Anonymous volunteers wrote in support of my presence in the Spirituality and Recovery groups on the Behavioral Health unit and local pastors sought out Board of Trustees members. I wrote letters of concern to the two representatives on the Board; the congregation where I am a member endorsed a massive letter-writing effort at its Congregational Meeting in January. To my knowledge, no one received a reply.

Into the mixture of feelings created by this traumatic experience, there appeared yet another event that now creates the context for me to describe my use of my own spirituality to cope. During her Christmas break, our college sophomore daughter brought home a refrigerator magnet with at once a simple and profound message. It is a quotation attributed to comedienne Gracie Allen that states, "Never place a period where God has placed a comma."

I reflect on this message as I continue living through what has become a lengthy "comma time" in my life and that of my family. There's a sermon about spirituality in that magnet. The comma, used in grammar to indicate a pause in a sentence, symbolizes the time of waiting and transition that my family and I continue to experience. For us, this comma time means:

- remembering God's nearness and waiting, pausing, listening, discerning, and quietly praying.
- diligently sending out my resume for full-time positions; going for interviews . . . declining some position offers, not being selected for others; calculating exactly when the last severance payment went into the bank.
- reflecting on the power of change in life. Change is a threat when it is done to me; it is an opportunity when I initiate it.

"Comma time" has also been a time of connectedness to an ecumenical placement agency where, since March 1, 1999, I have been a half-time interim chaplain to another local hospital. This hospital seeks clinically trained guidance and stability in their pastoral program consisting of eight local pastors who serve as volunteer on-call chaplains. There is also a desire by the hospital to increase the awareness of staff toward the value of pastoral care.

This part-time position has also been more "comma time" for me. I have never had a half time or an interim position before. I have taken on various limited roles as the interim–pastoral care provider as a one-person department manager, observer, consultant, supervisor of clergy volunteers, and preparer for "the permanent."

In these months since the "bomb" dropped, I have experienced the same feelings with which I have helped patients, families, and staff: anger, disbelief, fear, depression, denial, bitterness, betrayal, loneliness, self-pity. . . . In over 24 years of congregational and hospital ministry I have helped them express and validate these feelings. I knew the horror stories I had heard others tell at national pastoral care meetings, but now I have experienced them too.

Looking back on my journey, I am able to reflect on several "learnings" that might assist others when they face similar news:

- The hospital's cost reduction decision did not impact only me. My wife and children have experienced many feelings parallel to those I faced. We have attempted to cope with the on-going stress through increased exercise, asking more directly how each other is doing, and a greater focus on discerning what are the really important components to our relationships.

- In reviewing my Myers-Briggs personality type (ISFJ), I am more mindful of my tendency to "awfulize" things and fall victim to self-pity, of my tendency to move against what challenges me. In response, I seek and absorb glimpses of hope, whether spoken to me by others or encountered in times of prayer and meditation.

- Loyalty ain't what it used to be! The "bottom line" rules the business decision-making processes. My colleague and I chuckle at the realization that the reduction of our "enormous salaries" must have enabled the hospital to balance its budget.

- I am truly blessed with connections–family, friends, former co-workers, congregations, and Association relationships; networking means that I am not going through this process alone, although at first that is all I could feel.

- The hospital arranged for my colleague and me to receive the services of a professional "Outplacement and Career Search" agency. This support has been helpful in my search process; however, in cynical moments I wonder how the hospital can afford them if they cannot afford two chaplains.

I personally know that God's presence is most real when illness, loss, emotional turmoil or other disruptions punctuate life. The gift of hope, witnessed to every day by my wife and children, serves to remind me of God's grace, reminds me simply to live and to trust day-by-day. This is God's quietest intervention, but perhaps the one used most often.

How Has Health Care Reform
Affected Professional Chaplaincy Programs
and How Are Department Directors
Responding?

Larry VandeCreek, DMin, BCC

SUMMARY. No published studies were identified that describe the impact of health care reform on professional chaplaincy departments in hospital settings. Results from a random sample (N = 370) of department directors indicate that 45 percent report no budgetary consequences, 27 percent have experienced budgetary cutbacks, and 17 percent describe departmental growth. The cutbacks most often involve the loss of staff chaplain positions. Directors also describe past and future strategies for resisting downsizing trends. *[Article copies available for a fee from The Haworth Document Delivery Service: 1-800-342-9678. E-mail address: <getinfo@haworth pressinc.com> Website: <http://www.haworthpressinc.com>]*

KEYWORDS. Clergy, chaplain, pastoral counseling, pastoral care, health care reform

Most chaplains believe that health care reform poses a significant threat to their ministry. Even those programs in religiously affiliated institutions are not exempt. The executive director of the NACC (Dris-

---

Larry VandeCreek is Director, Department of Pastoral Research, The HealthCare Chaplaincy, Inc., New York, NY.

Address correspondence to: Larry VandeCreek, The HealthCare Chaplaincy, 307 East 60th Street, New York, NY 10022-1505.

[Haworth co-indexing entry note]: "How Has Health Care Reform Affected Professional Chaplaincy Programs and How Are Department Directors Responding?" VandeCreek, Larry. Co-published simultaneously in *Journal of Health Care Chaplaincy* (The Haworth Pastoral Press, an imprint of The Haworth Press, Inc.) Vol. 10, No. 1, 2000, pp. 7-17; and: *Professional Chaplaincy: What Is Happening to It During Health Care Reform?* (ed: Larry VandeCreek) The Haworth Pastoral Press, an imprint of The Haworth Press, Inc., 2000, pp. 7-17. Single or multiple copies of this article are available for a fee from The Haworth Document Delivery Service [1-800-342-9678, 9:00 a.m. - 5:00 p.m. (EST). E-mail address: getinfo@haworth pressinc.com].

coll, 1999) stated, "Some of the most endangered settings for chaplains are the 'Catholic' ones."

Clearly, professional chaplaincy needs a comprehensive study from a representative sample of department directors who, together, can begin to answer the question, "What's happening to us?" In this section, we report results from such a study by describing how we selected a sample of directors, the questionnaire we sent them, and the quantitative results. Narratives about downsizing experiences written by the Directors as part of their questionnaire responses are found in the next section.

METHODS

The Selection of Department Directors

Information was gathered from a representative sample of professional chaplaincy department directors because the results would then be relevant to the entire field. This mandated a random sample and deliberate selection processes for each of the three major organizations. A brief but detailed description of these processes is necessary to encourage confidence in the results.

As regards the Association of Professional Chaplains (then the College of Chaplains and the Association of Mental Health Clergy), participants were identified in two steps. First, listings in the Directory that described the chaplain as "Director" or some similar category were identified. Second, the names in the most recent "One Person Pastoral Care Department" specialty group were used because such chaplains would not likely be listed as the leader of a department. A random sample of participants was drawn after duplications, students, and retired chaplains were dropped from these two lists.

The National Association of Catholic Chaplains provided their mailing list containing department directors. A random sample was drawn from it after crossing off the names of Canadian directors.

The ACPE Directory was used to construct that list. Contact with its Regional Directors determined whether a supervisor was the department director and a random sample was chosen from the resultant list. These three random samples were then organized by state; names of individuals and programs were compared and duplicates eliminated. Having judged that a total sample of 500 department directors was adequate, the final mailing list contained 154 names drawn from the membership of the College of Chaplains and Association of Mental Health Clergy, 179 from ACPE, and 167 from the National Association of Catholic Chaplains. While these totals were not exactly equal, some of these participants held dual memberships and could be counted as part of at least two groups.

The Questionnaire

In the questionnaire, we asked for information concerning departmental changes during the previous ten years and what they anticipated in the future. In addition to a wide range of inquiries about department characteristics, we also listed 14 strategies that the Director potentially used in the past and could use in the future to combat the threat of downsizing. The last questionnaire item asked Directors to write a narrative about their experience with downsizing and ideas as to what the field of professional chaplaincy could do about it.

The Process

We contracted with a printing company to produce questionnaire booklets. We coded the mailing lists and the booklets so that we could contact those who did not respond and created personally addressed, signed cover letters, mailing these materials along with a postage-paid return envelope. The cover letter urged those who were not in administrative positions to forward the questionnaire. One week later we sent a postcard to all participants that thanked those who had responded and reminded others to complete the questionnaire. Two weeks later we sent a second packet of materials to non-responders with a new cover letter urging them to respond. As a result of these efforts, 430 department directors (86%) responded, 370 of whom (74%) provided usable information. The 12 percent who provided unusable results included some whom had left the administration of the department and others whose responses were incomplete.

Respondents represented the field of professional chaplaincy in a fairly equal manner. In broad geographic terms, they represented the Eastern (25%), Southern (25%), Midwestern (36%), and Western (14%) regions of the U.S. The primary organizational affiliation claimed by department directors included ACPE (30%), APC (35%), and NACC (30%). An approximately equal percentage of Directors represented institutions of various sizes. For example, 18 percent reported the institution size as 100 patients or less; 26 percent were employed by hospitals with a census of 101 to 200 patients. Institutions with a daily of census of 201 to 300 patients employed 19 percent of the department heads and 15 percent of the respondents described institutions of 301-400 patients. Twenty-two percent reported that they worked in hospitals with 401 or more patients. These characteristics regarding region, professional identity, and institution size strengthens the assumption that the results are representative of the field of professional chaplaincy.

RESULTS

Department Directors indicated whether and how health care reform had impacted the Department. As described in Table 1, the largest percentage of Departments (45%) reported that it had not made budgetary differences. A substantial number of programs (27%), however, reported budgetary cutbacks. Interestingly, 17 percent reported that it contributed to Department growth.

Another item asked Directors to describe what they lost if downsizing took place (Table 2). Here it was evident that, when downsizing occurred, personnel were lost most frequently, including staff chaplain (28%) and support positions (19%). The results suggest that often Directors lost budget money and had to make a decision concerning cutbacks themselves (25%).

Since Departments reported a variety of experiences with reform efforts (Table 1), it was important to identify associated institutional

TABLE 1. How Has Health Care Reform Impacted Pastoral Care Departments?

Percent	N	Department Impact
45	168	It has not made any budgetary differences up to the present time
27	99	It has caused budget cutbacks
17	63	It has contributed to growth in the Department (i.e., increased budget, staffing et al.)
4	15	It has contributed to other difficulties

Note: Total N = 370 respondents; Seven percent (N = 25) did not respond to the item. This table reports responses to a questionnaire item with five response categories. "It has not made any budgetary differences up to the present time" above also contains responses to "It has not made any budgetary differences . . . but more productivity is expected."

TABLE 2. When Downsizing Occurred, How Did It Effect Departments?

Percent	N	Department Impact
28	104	Lost staff chaplain positions
25	94	Lost budget money–Department decided where to make cuts
19	69	Lost staff support positions
15	56	Lost opportunity to add new positions
11	40	Lost space
9	34	Lost CPE stipends
9	34	Other miscellaneous impacts
9	32	No salary increases for most Department employees
6	21	Not lost support positions, but cannot add new support
2	8	Decreased salary for staff or CPE positions

Note: Respondents checked as many items as applied and this compounds the totals.

and departmental characteristics. That is, were there characteristics consistently associated with the responses? A wide variety of institutional and organizational characteristics as reported in the questionnaire were examined to answer this question. The information in Table 3 reports these variables and the results. Two characteristics emerged as significant–the number of chaplain FTEs and the presence of a CPE program in the Department. It is noteworthy that none of the other variables in the table were significantly influential.

The influence of Department size (FTEs) on the experience of downsizing is evident in Table 4. The way to interpret these results is to note that if Department size is not a factor in the effects of reform efforts, the percentages in the two rows across the columns would be approximately equal. It would not make a significant difference if the Department were smaller (in the Table, less than 3.0 FTEs) or larger (3.0 FTE chaplains or more) nor would the percentage vary according to the impact of reform efforts as represented in the column headings. As a matter of fact, however, Department size does make a significant difference. The first column describes department size for those Directors who reported no budgetary effect of reform efforts and approximate 60-40-percentage split exists according to department size. That approximate division is also found in column four. But the divisions for those who reported budget cuts (column 2) and growth (column 3) are very different. In both instances, the column percentages for those who report budget cuts and growth display a 40-60-percentage split. Thus, it becomes clear that the number of FTE chaplains in the department is significantly related to the impact of reform. It means that

TABLE 3. Institution/Department Characteristics and Their Association to the Impact of Health Care Reform

Institution/Department Characteristics	Association
1. The regional location of the Institution	(−)
2. The type of Institution (i.e., general hospital, psychiatric hospital et al.)	(−)
3. The Institution's size (i.e., average daily census)	(−)
4. Whether the Institution was religiously affiliated	(−)
5. Whether professional chaplaincy had departmental status	(−)
6. The administrative level to which the Department Director reported	(−)
7. The frequency with which the Director reported to a new administrator	(−)
8. Whether the Director believed that the faith stance of the Administrator was important	(−)
9. The number of chaplain positions funded by the institution (FTEs)	(+)
10. The number of chaplain positions funded outside the Institution's budget	(−)
11. The percentage of departmental ministry provided by volunteer chaplains	(−)
12. The amount of administrative experience possessed by the Department Director	(−)
13. The length of time the Director had responsibility for the Department	(−)
14. The primary professional identity reported by the Department Director	(−)
15. The presence of a CPE program in the Department	(+)
16. The percentage of outpatient ministry provided by the Department	(−)

Note: These results are produced by a Univariate Polychotomous Logistic Regression Analysis which examines response patterns between the categories described in Table 1 (i.e., impact of reform efforts on departments) and the characteristics listed in this Table. The Department's experience with downsizing was coded as follows: 1 = has contributed to Department growth; 2 = not made any budgetary differences; 3 = not made any budgetary differences, but more productivity is expected; 4 = has caused budget cutbacks. (+) indicates a statistically significant relationship ($p < .05$). Positive relationships (+) exist between all four of these experiences of the downsizing threat and the number of chaplain FTEs as well as the presence of a CPE program (details in Tables 4 and 5).

larger departments lost resources more often than smaller departments, but the results also make it clear that larger departments were also more often likely to grow. This is puzzling evidence that merits additional examination. It means that, given health care reform efforts, some larger departments grew while others suffered cutbacks. This suggests hidden, influential variables that are not evident in these results. We will return to this concern later.

In Table 5 the results concerning the influence of CPE programs on the impact of health care reform are reported. Once again, those departments that describe no budgetary effect are divided in an approximate 60-40 split concerning whether they contain a CPE program. Departments without CPE programs tend to report no budgetary effects. And once again, departments that report budget cuts and growth are the reverse–they tend to be those with CPE programs. Once again, these results suggest hidden variables that would explain why both budget cuts and growth are reported by departments with CPE programs.

TABLE 4. The Association Between Department FTEs and the Impact of Health Care Reform

FTEs	Impact of Health Care Reform				
	No Effect N (%)	Budget Cuts N (%)	Produced Growth N (%)	Other Difficulties N (%)	Totals N
0.5-2.9	95 (58%)	35 (37%)	24 (38%)	9 (64%)	163
3.0 or more	69 (42%)	60 (63%)	39 (62%)	5 (36%)	173
Totals	164	95	63	14	336

Notes: N = number of Department Directors; percents apply to column data. Statistical differences determined by Chi Square: DF = 4; Value = 15.20; p = 0.004. The significant differences in these results are most easily seen by comparing percentages across columns. Note that the larger percentage in each column varies by FTEs per Department.

TABLE 5. The Association Between Presence of Departmental CPE Program and the Impact of Health Care Reform

CPE Program	No Effect N (%)	Budget Cuts N (%)	Produced Growth N (%)	Other Difficulties N (%)	Totals N
No	101 (62%)	44 (46%)	25 (40%)	7 (50%)	177
Yes	63 (38%)	52 (54%)	37 (60%)	7 (50%)	159
Totals	164	96	62	14	336

Note: N = number of Department directors; percentages apply to column totals. Results in the Totals column may differ from those in Table 4 because of missing data. Statistical differences determined by Chi Square: DF = 4; Value = 14.18; p = 0.007. The significant differences in these results are most easily seen by comparing percentages across columns. Note that the larger percentage in each column varies by FTEs per Department.

The questionnaire also asked Directors to indicate what they expected as regards the threats of reform in the future. They indicated (Table 6) an expectation that "the threat of cutbacks will increase" (41%). Some (28%) expected the threat to decrease and these may be at least some of the Directors who already suffered cutbacks and thus believe that they have paid the price. More than one-fourth of the Directors acknowledged that they did not know what to expect.

A section of the questionnaire listed 15 potential strategies the Directors may have used in the past and present to defend against the threats of downsizing. They were instructed to divide 100 percent of their strategies among these categories and the results (Table 7) indicated that cultivating positive relationships with decision-makers was used by 81 percent of the Department Directors. Additionally, this strategy constituted the largest mean percentage of all strategies (12.5% of the 100% used by all Directors when taken as an aggregate).

Another section focused on future responses to the threat of down-

TABLE 6. What Do Department Directors Anticipate as Regards the Future?

Percent	N	Anticipated Department Impact
41	152	The threat of cutbacks will increase
28	105	The threat of cutbacks will decrease
26	94	Uncertain

Note: Five percent (N = 19) did not respond to this questionnaire item.

TABLE 7. Past and Current Strategies of Directors in Response to the Threats of Health Care Reform

Rank	% Depts That Used the Strategy*	Range of Percentages Reported**	Mean Percent***	Item Content
1	81	0.1-100	12.5	Cultivate positive relationships with decision makers
2	77	1.0-90	11.9	Develop strong involvements in interdisciplinary care
3	72	1.0-95	8.1	Take responsibility for additional activities
4	70	0.5-75	8.7	Build community support for the Department
5	67	0.5-85	7.6	Build advocates among powerful non-administrative persons who will fight for the Department
6	64	0.5-100	8.1	Let decision-makers know that patients/families/staff need and appreciate an internally funded dept.
7	64	0.5-100	9.9	Document all pastoral care visits in the chart
8	62	1.0-90	6.6	Build/maintain a strong presence in development of institutional policies
9	62	0.5-100	5.6	Communicate directly with physicians about difficult cases with which the chaplain is working
10	39	2.0-40	3.4	Develop case studies and statistics to support the Department
11	32	0.5-25	2.5	Voluntarily cut back in less essential areas
12	30	1.0-85	2.5	Conduct research that demonstrates the contribution of the Department
13	22	1.0-50	2.8	Focus on fund-raising for the Department from other sources
14	18	1.0-100	3.9	Other strategies
15	11	1.0-100	1.7	Do little to protect staff, space and budget

Note: N = 370. Respondents divided 100 percent of their strategies among the 15 categories. *Indicates the percentage of Directors who attributed any percentage to the strategy. **Indicates the range of percentages reported by Directors. ***Indicates the mean percentage from all those reported. Item contents quote those listed in the questionnaire.

sizing and presented these same strategies. It asked Directors to indicate their use of these strategies should the threat of downsizing continue. These results (Table 8) create an interesting comparison to the importance given to strategies used in the past. The past and future importance of seven strategies are contrasted in Table 9. Directors in the future will depend less on cultivating positive relationships with institutional decision makers and more on bringing pressure to bear on them by way of pointing out the needs and appreciation of patients/families/staff as well as using non-administrative advocates including community support.

TABLE 8. Future Strategies of Directors in Response to the Threats of Health Care Reform

Rank	% Depts That Used the Strategy*	Range of Percentages Reported**	Mean Percent***	Item Content
1	56	0.5-100	9.6	Communicate further with decision makers about how patients/families/staff need and appreciate an internally funded Department
2	55	0.5-50	8.1	Call on advocates among powerful non-administrative persons to fight for the Department
3	54	2.0-50	8.8	Build community support for the Department that will positively influence institutional decision makers
4	52	2.0-100	8.5	Cultivate additional positive relationships with decision makers
5	47	2.0-50	6.7	Find additional research demonstrating the Department's contribution
6	44	2.0-65	5.8	Increase interdisciplinary involvements
7	41	1.0-70	6.2	Take responsibility for additional activities
8	37	2.0-100	5.9	Document pastoral care in patient charts more thoroughly
9	37	2.0-100	4.3	Increase communication with physicians about difficult cases with which chaplains are working
10	37	1.0-100	7.8	Focus on fund-raising for the Department from other sources
11	34	2.0-50	4.4	Develop more case studies and statistics to support the Department
12	33	2.0-40	3.8	Increase departmental presence in institutional policy decisions
13	20	0.5-100	2.4	Voluntarily cut back in less essential areas
14	15	0.5-100	4.7	Other
15	7	2.0-100	3.9	Cannot do anything more

Note: N = 370. Respondents divided 100 percent of their strategies among the 15 categories. *Indicates the percentage of Directors who attributed any percentage to the strategy. **Indicates the range of percentages reported by Directors. ***Indicates the mean percentage from all those reported. Item contents quote those listed in the questionnaire.

TABLE 9. Comparison of Past/Present and Future Strategies

Past/Present Rank	Future Rank	Strategy Content
1	4	Cultivate positive relationships with institutional decision makers
2	6	Increase interdisciplinary involvements
3	7	Take responsibility for additional activities
4	3	Build community support for the Department that will positively influence institutional decision makers
5	2	Call on advocates among powerful non-administrative persons to fight for the Department
6	1	Communicate further with decision makers about how patients/families/staff need and appreciate an internally funded department
12	5	Find additional research demonstrating the Department's contribution

DISCUSSION

This appears to be the first published study that examines the impact of health care reform on professional chaplaincy departments in hospitals. Selected results are briefly discussed.

First, the response rate to the questionnaire is very high. While the professional appearance of the materials and follow-up efforts likely influenced the response rate, it may also indicate that Directors felt such a study was needed. The results seem reliable because of the large number of department directors in the sample representing all geographic regions. Department and hospital sizes also vary.

These results provide evidence that can stabilize rumors and fantasies about the impact of health care reform. The results suggest that, although increased scrutiny is prevalent, nearly a majority of the departments (45%) suffered no budgetary reductions. It is likely that nursing and allied health departments have fared worse. And, as regards pastoral care departments, changes have brought bane and blessing, personnel reductions and growth. The most frequent form taken by downsizing is the loss of staff chaplain positions and these losses are related to department size and the presence of a CPE program. Here the contradictory findings noted in regards to Table 1 become more evident. Clearly, some variables not included in the questionnaire are active. This motivated further research which is addressed in the article by Lucas which appears in this volume.

The results concerning strategies (Tables 7, 8, and 9) clarify how department directors have engaged reform efforts. The rankings in

Tables 7 and 8 suggest that directors attempt to make departments more valuable to the institutions by building good-will with administrators and adopting additional responsibilities. There has been relatively little interest in seeking funding beyond the institution and Tables 8 and 9 suggest that it will likely not become an attractive option.

The materials in Table 9 suggest shifting strategies. These changes likely occur as directors learn what works bests–and what has not worked. The ranking of the future strategies seems to suggest that directors will increasingly turn to placing pressure on administration rather than appealing to their good will.

In summary, health care reform is here to stay. It has raised the anxiety of everyone and accurate information is a helpful remedy to fantasy and fear. The results suggest that a similar study in the future is needed to identify the changing influences of reform efforts.

REFERENCE

Driscoll, J. 1999. "Putting a spin on chaplaincy." *Vision* (February), 5.

Health Care Reform:
Analysis of Narrative Responses
from Directors of Pastoral Care Departments

M. Patrice McCarthy, PhD, RN

SUMMARY. This paper is a narrative analysis of comments written by hospital pastoral care department directors in response to the questionnaire item that asked them to write about their experience with health care reform and to make suggestions as to what the profession could do about it. Three central themes included: (1) the importance of and need for administrative support of the department, (2) the importance of departmental visibility within the institution, and (3) the challenges of embracing change. Two secondary themes were the admonishing of peer department directors concerning inadequate performance and the ministry to hospital staff during reform efforts. *[Article copies available for a fee from The Haworth Document Delivery Service: 1-800-342-9678. E-mail address: <getinfo@haworthpress inc.com> Website: <http://www.haworthpressinc.com>]*

KEYWORDS. Clergy, chaplain, pastoral counseling, pastoral care, health care reform

This paper identifies themes in the narratives written by Pastoral Care Department Directors as they participated in the questionnaire project described above. These narratives constituted their responses

Address correspondence to: M. Patrice McCarthy, MedCentral College of Nursing, 335 Glefsner Avenue, Mansfield, OH 44903.

The author gratefully acknowledges the assistance of Mary Ellen Kelley, RN, MSN, MEd, and doctoral candidate, in the analysis of the data for this article.

[Haworth co-indexing entry note]: "Health Care Reform: Analysis of Narrative Responses from Directors of Pastoral Care Departments." McCarthy, M. Patrice. Co-published simultaneously in *Journal of Health Care Chaplaincy* (The Haworth Pastoral Press, an imprint of The Haworth Press, Inc.) Vol. 10, No. 1, 2000, pp. 19-36; and: *Professional Chaplaincy: What Is Happening to It During Health Care Reform?* (ed: Larry VandeCreek) The Haworth Pastoral Press, an imprint of The Haworth Press, Inc., 2000, pp. 19-36. Single or multiple copies of this article are available for a fee from The Haworth Document Delivery Service [1-800-342-9678, 9:00 a.m. - 5:00 p.m. (EST). E-mail address: getinfo@haworthpressinc.com].

19

to the final item that asked them to describe their experiences with and/or their anxieties about downsizing. They were also asked to include ideas about what professional chaplaincy can or ought to do during this era of reform.

My training is in phenomenological qualitative research and typically the purpose is to describe the nature of "a lived experience" based on interview materials. The final product of such an analysis is a metaphor or statement of "the unity of meaning" discovered from within the verbatim descriptions of the experience. The language of this unity of meaning is derived from the researcher's engagement in a dialectical/dialogical process of deep reflection about the descriptions provided by research participants.

A formal phenomenological analysis was neither feasible nor appropriate here because the data consisted of written comments to a questionnaire item rather than a personal interview. Since such a discussion did not occur, my approach reflected the spirit of the phenomenological tradition by remaining true to the language of the participants. No effort was made to derive a unity of meaning that captured the essence of the downsizing experience.

In the qualitative analysis process, attention is given to meanings and understandings of experiences rather than frequency of data in the material. In the first step, I read all the narratives for global impressions and then again a number of times for more specificity. The language of the respondents was then used as a basis for reflection to identify descriptive categories that characterized the issues delineated in the responses. These categories were then reviewed to identify possible interpretations of the responses. In the last step, direct quotations were identified to illustrate the actual content of the categories. These categories emerged apart from any knowledge on my part of the quantitative findings reported above.

The comments from respondents ranged in length from one or two sentences to multiple pages. By far, the most typical response was two to four brief paragraphs. All responses were included in the first analysis. The size and type of institution was then used to classify subsets of responses. These included faith-based and non-faith-based community hospitals. The responses were then reread for distinctions among the issues and to examine the potential influence of affiliative status to issues identified in the global review process.

FINDINGS

The narratives reflected three primary categories: (1) the importance of and need for administrative support of the department, (2) the importance of departmental visibility within the institution, and (3) the challenges of embracing change. Two secondary themes were also identified. They were (1) the admonishing of peer department directors concerning inadequate performance and (2) the ministry to hospital staff. Each is discussed below.

The Importance of and Need for Administrative Support

This concern dominated the responses. The narratives indicated both the complexity and extent of influence that administrative support has on the very identity and nature of the pastoral care ministry and those who provide it. One prominent aspect of administrative support was the perceived or actual value of pastoral care to the institution as well as its relevance to patient care. The responses concerning administrative support were both positive and negative but almost always reflected its crucial role. For example, one Director wrote:

> Due to the almost 30 years of chaplaincy at the hospital, the chaplaincy is a strong, viable aspect of treatment. The support of the VP whom the chaplain reports to is essential . . . Downsizing has created remarkable changes in the agency . . . The chaplaincy department is expected now to cover the whole network (of 22 agencies). Yet, there are administrators who would not think twice about cutting the whole program. (Chaplain ID # 9.1003)

Another department director wrote:

> The current hospital administration is not supportive of pastoral care services or spiritual care–they say they are but actions show otherwise. A main problem is that they have their own paradigm of what pastoral care is based on (their) experiences of (it) years ago. . . . (79;3386)

A prominent aspect of administrative support was the Director's perception of the values held by administrative persons. They were regarded as central to decisions about the department, including the organizational placement and duties that were assigned to it. The following three responses represented this theme.

> I believe we are going through a knee jerk reaction of finances related to a recent merger. The administrator is taking this opportunity to do something to the spiritual care program of our institution that he has really wanted to do for a long time and it really has no connection to the finances. (285;3448)

> At our hospital the threat has been more related to the rise or fall in revenue or perceived threats of that. The person I report to has been very supportive–(perhaps) because of her own nursing background and commitment to total care. (303;1071)

> Some of my suspicions about the reasons for cuts in pastoral care include the fact that the CEO is Roman Catholic and has a limited understanding of pastoral care. We have had CPE here for 24 years and the hospital relied on students and volunteers for a significant part of pastoral care. (262;1106)

Many of the participants blamed their administrators for the downsizing. They perceived the administrators to be businessmen with limited understanding of the value of their ministry within the hospital community. For example:

> The changes have been intense; especially the downsizing that has taken place as health care has become more a business than a ministry (especially as health care senior management is now consisting of lay leadership). This becomes more complicated (and) involved as frequently their faith may be radically different and they themselves are new to health care (i.e., coming from banks, etc.). (2;3401)

The dissonance between the value of ministry as perceived by pastoral care providers in comparison to administrators was at the heart of the anxiety. The formal religion of the Administrator, the personal relationship between the Administrator and the Director were regarded as very important as well as the patient demands for pastoral services. One Director wrote:

> The faith community of the top administrative persons is an important factor in the survival of pastoral care–if such a faith

committed person is not in those positions; it is vital to be able to demonstrate cost-effectiveness of pastoral care. (13;1065)

Another way in which Administrator-Director relationships came into focus involved the structural position and reporting relationships within the institution as well as the scope of responsibilities that came under the rubric of pastoral care. The shift of pastoral care from a freestanding department to a component of social services or as an overseer of hospital volunteers reflected institutional values.

The breadth of the support for pastoral care both within and beyond the institution was also critical to the concern about the future. Even in the face of supportive administrators, the scope of community support for pastoral care lessened the degree of anxiety about the future. For those highly anxious about the impact of a single person in an administrative position, building a base of support beyond institutional confines was cited as a means to ensure a viable future.

> Twice over the past 2-3 years, administration (Board of Directors) has sought to eliminate the position and department of chaplains. Both times they met with fierce community support for the department. (220;2252)

In the analysis, distinctions between faith-based and non-faith-based community hospitals were sought. It was anticipated that considerable differences in values and administrative support would exist. While I found some differences, they were not as distinct as I anticipated. The following three comments reflected a diversity in the Catholic institutions themselves.

> I feel quite blessed at being in a Catholic health system that prioritizes spiritual care. If spiritual care is significantly downsized in our system, the sponsors will probably reconsider sponsorship. Spiritual care is the hallmark of our system and mission. (189;3352)

In contrast, note the following:

> My hospital is Catholic but we visit all denominations. Pastoral care doesn't seem to be that important to the institution. Sometimes I feel the administration doesn't know we exist. (91;3321)

Or again:

> I believe that although administrators think they understand spiritual care, in reality they often do not. In my experience, many administrators in Catholic facilities equate spiritual care with sacramental care. Thus, a priest is deemed necessary for good care; everything else is extra. It is, therefore, easy to cut positions for chaplains and keep positions for priest chaplains. (294;3362)

Even when pastoral care was defined as a central feature of the institution's mission, the issue of administrative support remained a concern for those in both faith-based and non-faith-based institutions. How can this be interpreted? The first obvious explanation is that, regardless of mission, all institutions have felt fiscal challenges and the need to respond to economic realities. Another plausible explanation is the influence of new, large networks comprised of institutions that were historically distinct in both mission and fiscal control. This new entity is now integrated in a way that challenges the survival of the faith-based mission. The following quote from a respondent in a faith-based institution captures the complexity of administrative support and the concern about the influence of the collaborating institutions.

> The only factor saving the department is the CEO's conviction, along with the sponsoring congregation, that the religious character of the acute care hospital is preserved through the maintenance of chaplaincy services. I believe the non-religious business minded VP's would down size the department in different ways because they publicly state the department represents overhead. Thus the department is more funded by the foundation which raises funds for chaplaincy, AIDS, hospice, etc., as part of the hospital to provide services to the community. If our system is absorbed into (another faith-based system) I will automatically lose my position, (the other) chaplain will manage the department and will report to a VP who knows nothing about pastoral care. (288;3467)

The Importance of Departmental Visibility Within the Institution

A second prominent issue concerned the degree of visibility of pastoral care departments within the institutions. Comments spanned a continuum. Some feared that their department was invisible while others focused on demonstrating visibility within the institution. Some department directors described strategies they had implemented to improve visibility. Many wrote that JCAHO accreditation criteria possessed positive leverage in the creation of more visibility with hospital administration.

> Because of the positive regard JCAHO puts on spiritual care and its role in accreditation, I see the future as positive because of these expectations. If pastoral care is to do anything proactive it should be with JCAHO and the expectations of a multidisciplinary approach to pastoral care by certified professionals in all disciplines. (30;2307)

The intensity of concern about visibility issues varied widely. Some made self-deprecating remarks about the inability of some pastoral care colleagues to market the valuable contribution they made to quality patient care. Thus, one wrote:

> We have failed as a profession to document and market our own contributions. Many doubt they can be documented. (5;1061)

Some department directors were concerned about other professional disciplines usurping authority from pastoral care departments. The content for this often was the invisibility and inadequacy of pastoral care personnel.

> Some of us have abdicated studies of spirituality to medical and nursing personnel who have a poor conceptual base and poor theology who produce offensive studies that are invalid. Poor management and accountability plague administration in pastoral care. (5;1061)

However, the more prevalent responses related to the issue of institutional visibility came in the form of creative problem solving designed to unabashedly market the value of the services provided by Departments to hospitals and communities at large.

> Get involved with community benefit initiatives. Assume a role of primary liaison between hospital and the religious community. Bring faith and health together–Teach parish nurses and health

ministry outreach coordinators how to provide spiritual care. Start doing hard data outcome measurements that show the positive and vast impact that faith has on making life-long sustained behavior changes. Link the values of pastoral care service with reduced length of stay–reduced costs–we should unionize nationwide as pastoral caregivers and make a national outcry against this insanity. (356;2166)

The push among the Directors to increase the visibility of their departments highlighted the importance of relationships as the major empowering force. The development of a broad range of relationships allowed for varied input as well as a broad base of support, and avoided the powerlessness of isolation.

I could be wrong but I believe the bottom line is still the relationship the chaplain has with his colleagues, patients, relatives and staff. If this is in place, there will always be a place for the department of pastoral care. (163;2486)

Another department head wrote:

A very strong key factor in protecting Pastoral Care from downsizing was the relationship with the board of trustee members who reversed the administration's initial plan to downsize pastoral care. As Director I had provided significant pastoral care to several board members and their families. The board members and key community leaders effectively had administration leave pastoral care out of the downsizing. (148;2202)

In summary, the Directors believe that the influence of JCAHO is very helpful as regards visibility. As indicated by one respondent from a non-faith based institution in a 101-300 bed institution, the standards regarding spiritual care were the foundation of the decision to hire the first director of pastoral care in the 74-year history of the institution. While seen as an ally, JCAHO cannot insure the future of pastoral care. The suggestions regarding extenuation of the base of support for Pastoral Care include strengthening relationships both within the institution with administrative and medical staff as well as establishing foundations to fiscally support the ministry. Several respondents suggest extending the work of pastoral care into home health and other community and home-based services.

Particularly in this time of change, a discussion of the vision and value of pastoral care becomes vitally important during the reengineering work that is pervasive in the healthcare environment. The challenge is to look at the current system and to imagine a vision of pastoral care in the system that can be articulated as an essential element of patient care. The ability of pastoral care directors to articulate a clear vision with administrators influences how administration then structures the department within the institution.

The Challenge of Embracing Change

The third category concerned the attitude toward change and the experience of downsizing. The heart of this stance was a strong resolve to reframe the negative downsizing experience into a positive opportunity for growth.

> When I think about the effects of downsizing on our department, my initial reaction is, indeed, anxiety. But actually the overall effects of downsizing have in our place been mixed or possibly even more positive than negative . . . We need to always recognize that we are not alone in this challenging and often frustrating era . . . All services and departments are under scrutiny with regard to questions about whether they are essential and, if essential, whether we could be more productive and efficient. I believe we have to find a whole variety of ways to respond to the challenge. This has meant we need to be creative in our response and re-think what we are doing in pastoral care. (121;1096)

Another wrote:

> Downsizing was across the board, so pastoral care wasn't singled out! But, tightening has been helpful in that we've been forced to focus and prioritize what we do. (112;1001)

And again:

> I really enjoy my ministry in a complex metro regional setting of four medical centers with pastoral care programs. My main challenge is to find enough time to do what I want to do:
>
> - Be productive in relating and being friends to our administrative people at all levels (a strong use of people skills).
> - Raising money–This has happened by my request. The unexpected result has been the rise in stature of our departments

and administration. We are now players and not simply sitting around waiting to be taken care of.
- Letting people know what we have to give as chaplains. Finances are a strong link to survival; we must practice good stewardship with our Department monies and use them in new and creative ministries.

I am very optimistic about our future and see our program as continuing to grow. In many cases I believe downsizing can be averted by strong leadership and the promotion of pastoral care both within and outside the institution. (8;1090)

The influence of downsizing has precipitated consolidations and mergers with other institutions so that network services are diversified. Some directors experienced these changes as requiring both expansion and constraint.

Downsizing at our hospital is paradoxical. There has been downsizing financially and in terms of personnel. Yet on the other hand there has been expansion as the hospital extends the network of services in the system . . . The chaplain has worked closely with the hospital and community and church leaders to raise the funds so that full-time pastoral care can be maintained. (164;2181)

Another wrote:

I believe the creative partnering initiatives between pastoral care programs and local congregations holds some promise of retaining some positions . . . I believe it is inevitable that large chaplain departments will decline in size if managed care continues to have a hammer lock on delivery systems. In part, I also believe some downsizing is justified. Being able to document the value-added nature of services is also essential to stave off being pruned. My center has not done well at concretely measuring the value-added nature of our work. We have mountains of anecdotal evidence though. (128;1105)

Again:

I am advocating for challenge, change and growth. Sometimes I feel like a voice crying out in the desert. Education about the new paradigm has to take place on all levels. A great deal of struggling and questioning is taking place and will take place. Change is never easy, but change is a sign of growth. (233;3339)

Another dimension of the embracing change theme emerged as a measure of hope for the future. This hope was in the context of the growing appreciation for spiritually related issues in the general population as well as in the formal health care system of providers.

Downsizing is primarily due to the economic crisis brought on by health care excesses for diagnosis and therapy. At the same time there is a significant interest in natural and alternative medicine and renewed awareness of the value of spiritual assessment/treatment. I fully expect the new demands for changes in health care will eventually include a new identity for pastoral care as part of the clinical pathways. I think the need for pastoral caregivers will increase and thus also increase the need for good CPE programs. (126;1022)

Another wrote:

With the encouragement and help of my VP, we have just completed preparation and have actually started a three-year program of spiritual enrichment for all employees and physicians. (241;3464)

And again:

If the accumulating evidence of the economic value of spiritual care is recognized by the government (besides NIH) and insurance, perhaps there will be an increased support of pastoral care, in-patient and outpatient. (215;2484)

During recovery from the trauma of downsizing, participants reported going through a grieving process for each real and perceived loss. The extent of the loss included one's own position or those of coworkers, relationships to administrators and interdisciplinary colleagues, and perhaps, most profoundly, a sense that the profession itself was being compromised.

I am anxious about my co-workers. I know I can probably keep my job but I can't be sure I can keep theirs. I am very anxious about mergers and takeovers. We are still a freestanding hospital, something of a dinosaur in health care. People here are very anxious about a hostile takeover. I had to work very hard to educate my immediate supervisor regarding pastoral care and the work and value of our department. My best allies are in the community. (15;1028)

Perhaps the most significant decision on the path from victim to survivor is to consciously grieve. Facilitating the grieving helps to preserve the will to care in a seemingly chaotic world.

I believe there is a serious loss of the meaning of work that is rewarding and enriching to the soul. People are putting in their time, they are tired and weary, and they are going home with no energy left for families or themselves. I have tried to help folks rekindle the meaning in their work by asking them why they do what they do. As they relate how they got into the field, sometimes the spark returns in their eyes. I believe there is a great deal of grief work to do involving individuals whose work has been building a department over the years only to have it dismantled. Re-framing that their work still remained good for the time it existed and that it stands on its own in memory as a monument to their effort. I have spoken to my administrator about the necessity of rituals to give thanks to those who have lost their jobs rather than simply having them depart without notice because to acknowledge them would be to admit the things we would not like to face. (24;2185)

Many Directors described their need to reach out to one another for comfort and support in order to complete their grieving process. Participation in small groups encouraged participants to identify with others and to realize that they are not alone. The group experience served as an effective buffer when denial was abandoned to expose the stark truth about downsizing. Group work curbed the negative coping behaviors of blame and victimization. When the group was able to confront downsizing head on for what it was, minus all the images that the mere mention of the word evokes, then the experience was described by many as an opportunity for personal and professional growth.

If I might, what we surely need in pastoral care is not investment in anxiety about downsizing so much as a compelling functional programmatic conception of what pastoral care can, should and needs to be doing in our communities and institutions of care. That may be effective in capturing the attention and financial investment of those who hold the purse strings of these institutions and governmental agencies. If we're not getting the bucks, maybe its because we ain't doing the job; and I don't mean just immediate pastoral care on the one to one, but pastoral care to agencies and their planning. I (am referring to) developing a national profile that calls people's attention to what we do, and why it works, and what else it can do. I am looking to you guys as well as myself for the answers as to how to do this. It concerns me that one of the first things that come out of our new offices is a concern about fighting downsizing. This sounds rather parochial and self-serving. It seems to me that it's been precisely the lack of a national, politically sophisticated, and socially progressive philosophy that has left us behind the times and found us last in line for the financial support we need to turn this society around. How about it? (125;1016)

The anxiety associated with downsizing persisted as a powerful emotive force and challenge even in institutions whose mission called for particular attention to pastoral needs of patients and families.

Words like 'freeze' automatically create anxiety and intense strategizing opportunities. I have had to 'strategize' myself into not capitulating to lesser quality/credentials, i.e., move to replace a CPE supervisor with a lesser paid/credited staff chaplain. I have found our department increasing in supervisory positions and residency programs as I have managed my anger and stayed faithful to my vision and commitment to a strong CPE driven pastoral ministry. The key for me is also to rely in our hospital's faith based mission and leadership. (113;1130)

In summary, the challenge of change called for departments to be creative in providing care. It was clear that some met this challenge more directly than others; some seemed overwhelmed and found it difficult to see the implicit opportunities.

Important Secondary Themes

Two themes merit attention here, namely: (1) the admonishing of peer department heads and (2) the need to minister to hospital staff members. They were secondary because they lacked the urgency attributed to the need for administrative support, department visibility, and the challenge of embracing change. Nonetheless, they were clearly important to Directors.

Admonishing Peer Department Directors

While comments critical of pastoral care practitioners were infrequent, they did represent a voice of concern. Some of these comments have already been quoted above. The admonitions pertained to the adequacy of preparation for leadership roles, contributions to research regarding impact on patient care, and the balance of graduates from training programs in relation to the number of positions available. The following six quotations represented the substance of these comments.

> The field of institutional pastoral care must develop better administrative training and encourage the development of a more adventuresome and entrepreneurial interest. We seem to have come full circle in the sense of early years when the health care institutions didn't fund our work and we had to secure it elsewhere to full funding to the current reaction of support. We must be more creative and develop alternative sources again. Many of our number pale at the thought. (205;1008)

> The field of pastoral care must move out of acute care settings of hospital and show relative contribution in community, this related to wellness and alternative therapy partnerships. Today's chaplains are too inflexible and not trained to provide leadership only to in-patient visitation. If we don't change pastoral care will die. (97;3360)

> Another contributing factor is the proliferation of CPE Programs. There is an over supply of people qualified to be chaplains and no jobs . . . There should be someone assessing the need for CPE programs and whether or not more supervisors should be trained. Positions for staff chaplains or directors in non-CPE hospitals are virtually non-existent. (178;2170)

> Much of the downsizing in institutions is because we have not been effective with what we have. We treat our positions like

"sacred cows." There was a lack of accountability. The person to whom I report is not out to ax the department. They want better use of our skills. We are moving out into the community, as we should be. (200;3442)

Downsizing is a painful reality. I believe we need to "sell" ourselves. Go public–speak out to the public. Let them know what is happening. Let the public realize we are body-mind-spirit-emotions and all need attention. My experience has been to witness Chaplains who were sterile reciting formulas. Hopefully these are being 'downsized.' (362;3332)

Research and good data demonstrating our contribution to the actual recovery and health of the patient is vital to keeping pastoral care. We do not articulate well our contribution to the actual physiological health of the patient even though we intuitively know the effect. (137;1108)

The issues identified in many of the above comments were summarized by one respondent's call for a programmatic conception of what pastoral care can, should and needs to be doing in communities and institutions of care. This sentiment captured the challenge of these comments by suggesting the need to re-evaluate the structural and facilitative role pastoral care plays in health care and how best to achieve its goal. One respondent suggested that the lack of "a national, politically sophisticated and socially progressive philosophy is responsible for pastoral care being behind the times and also last in line for financial support" (125;1016).

Ministry to Hospital Staff

The impact of downsizing on institutional administration and its employees was mentioned as an area of concern. Departmental integrity required that it supported not only patients and their family members but also the staff when downsizing struck. One Director wrote, "The department's reputation is upheld by what you are doing, not on what you did or will do" (77;3447). Models of staff care in down sizing situations integrated the Department into the fabric of the institution. Staff retreats and education about stress/pain reduction techniques of centering prayer, guided imagery, meditation chant, and energy work were identified as ways to accomplish this objective. The concern about morale in general was evident throughout the comments and contributed significantly to the issue of downsizing.

> The greatest frustration is the feeling and in many ways the expectation to minister to hurt staff who have been terminated and those who remain. If I ask to increase my department size I'm setting up the very real possibility of being downsized in the future. (44;2277)

Viewing the pastoral care department as a space that allowed for grieving the impact of downsizing and being a voice for the spirit of the institution was highlighted as a strategy for advocacy rather than adopting a guarded posture within the agency.

> As the Spiritual Care Staff continues to work here, we feel a special call not only to patients and their families. We seek to respond to the whole hospital staff which includes administrators, physicians, nurses and all who dedicate so much of their day to providing good health care in an ever changing world which so often only focuses on the negative. All in all, I feel we are called to walk daily in Faith and to model that to those we seek to serve. In this hospital, at this present time, Spiritual/Pastoral care is . . . ALIVE AND WELL! (370;2497)

DISCUSSION

The narratives make it clear that chaplains want to provide ministry within a humanistic, holistic framework in which spiritual growth can be nurtured. However, the perception is that managed care challenges and even assaults that framework. After more than a decade of downsizing, little evidence exists that a purely efficient approach maintains a competitive edge (Byrne, 1996). The traumatic, crisis environment created by downsizing profoundly affects chaplains within the hospital setting. The important question is whether the personal and professional losses are really necessary.

> Pastoral care has in my opinion become too focused on survival. Pastoral Care Departments are the last 'generalist' departments and need to be more prophetic and responsive. Downsizing is going to happen. The continuum of care is changing. Depart-

ments need to provide ministry to survivors of downsizing. I think as we have done this we have ingrained and blended ourselves tighter in the fabric of health care delivery in this system. We need to quit worrying about our survival and do that which we are called to do–fulfill our baptismal vows. The institution only gives us permission to function within its walls. It does not give us the power. (272;1122)

This sentiment supports the comments of many respondents who wish to move beyond the trauma of downsizing to reaffirm pastoral ministry as a profession that values the quality of life more highly than profit margin. Many comments refer to this ministry as a "calling" rather than a profession with financial motivations.

Personally I believe that the institutional churches ought to be supporting chaplaincy. However there is no strong history for this. It was only when health care institutions funded these positions that they flourished. But that provides a paradox with which I am not comfortable. Funded by the institution a chaplain's loyalty is to the institution and not to her/his faith. I do not want to say we are not to be accountable. Only that in being accountable we do not become a position that is easily interchangeable with any other position and does not have primary commitment to the divine. In a drive to prove the worth of chaplaincy in economic terms we must be careful lest we forget whom we represent. (27;2299)

While I don't mind working hard in spiritual care and education, I do not feel I want to put my energies into 'fighting' for my position or survival . . . Idealistic as it might sound I want to put my energy into spiritual ministry and not big business and its down-sizing. (189;3352)

In summary, this analysis sought to uncover central issues experienced by Directors of Pastoral Care Departments during health care reform efforts. While the concerns about these issues are prominent within the respondent's comments, it is also necessary to recognize the breadth of creative efforts undertaken by many in diverse institutions to strengthen their role and position. Across institutions of varying sizes and types, it is evident that considerable energy and creative attention is being focused on these matters.

While all of the issues identified here contain pragmatic implications, the underlying issues are the contrasting and often competing values. The conflict in values becomes manifest in a variety of ways. It may be evident within the institution itself or as a function of the fiscal challenges posed by reduced revenues as a result of the managed care model of reimbursement. The irony is that the limitations in funding occur just as the general public is calling for a renewed commitment to spiritual issues and as research findings are establishing a broader knowledge base about the significance of spiritual well-being as a contributor to overall health.

The current medically dominated health care arena bases its success and technological advances on a philosophy of science that by definition dismisses the relevance of metaphysics. By definition, spiritual beliefs, practices, and values are not 'knowable' as science and therefore are disregarded. As one respondent stated, "Pastoral care is not essential to medical care but is essential to health care" (14;1045). This statement exemplifies the distinction between old and new paradigms of thought. If pastoral care is thought of from an old paradigm perspective, it may never reach the prominence it deserves because it is not valued in that system of thought. We live, as Kolbenschlagg (1979) states, in a time of "the no longer and the not yet." That is, the old paradigm is clearly no longer adequate and a new paradigm has yet to pervade the consciousness of health care. Recognizing this context can free one's energies from old struggles (often experienced as personal devaluation) and focus them into creating new paradigms. The challenges are particularly poignant because pastoral care itself represents the very element denied as central to healing, health and wholeness. As a distinct practice, the field of pastoral care brings a unique knowledge to a creative dialogue about a new paradigm of hope and wholeness for society. Facing the challenges of this shift in paradigmatic thought will require clarity of vision and a discerning spirit on the journey.

REFERENCES

Byrne, J. (1996). Strategic planning. *Business Week*, August 26, pp. 45-51.
Kolbenschlagg, M. (1979). *Kiss sleeping beauty goodbye*. New York: Bantam Books.

Economic Rationalism and the Cost Efficiency of Hospital Chaplaincy: An Australian Study

Christopher Newell, PhD
Lindsay B. Carey, MAppSc

SUMMARY. Health care reform is also occurring in Australia and effects hospital chaplaincy programs. "Economic rationalism" is the philosophic foundation of this effort and its contrast with the values inherit in hospital chaplaincy are highlighted. Selected research results from the Australian system are described and the authors offer a perspective on the cost efficiency of hospital chaplaincy. *[Article copies available for a fee from The Haworth Document Delivery Service: 1-800-342-9678. E-mail address: <getinfo@haworthpressinc.com> Website: <http://www.haworthpressinc.com>]*

KEYWORDS. Clergy, chaplain, pastoral counseling, pastoral care, health care reform

INTRODUCTION: ECONOMICS AND CHAPLAINCY

Economic rationalism presents particular challenges for hospital chaplaincy throughout the Western world, including Australia. Indeed,

---

Christopher Newell is Senior Lecturer, School of Medicine, University of Tasmania, GPO Box 232-33, Hobart, Tasmania, Australia 7001 (E-mail: Christopher.Newell@utas.edu.au). Lindsay B. Carey is affiliated with the School of Public Health, La-Trobe University, Bundoora, Victoria, Australia 3083 (E-mail: Linz.Carey@latrobe.edu.au).

[Haworth co-indexing entry note]: "Economic Rationalism and the Cost Efficiency of Hospital Chaplaincy: An Australian Study." Newell, Christopher, and Lindsay B. Carey. Co-published simultaneously in *Journal of Health Care Chaplaincy* (The Haworth Pastoral Press, an imprint of The Haworth Press, Inc.) Vol. 10, No. 1, 2000, pp. 37-52; and: *Professional Chaplaincy: What Is Happening to It During Health Care Reform?* (ed: Larry VandeCreek) The Haworth Pastoral Press, an imprint of The Haworth Press, Inc., 2000, pp. 37-52. Single or multiple copies of this article are available for a fee from The Haworth Document Delivery Service [1-800-342-9678, 9:00 a.m. - 5:00 p.m. (EST). E-mail address: getinfo@haworthpressinc.com].

hospital chaplaincy currently exists in the face of a post-modern social system that suggests that economics can provide a solution and value system that will solve financial crises within the health care system. Thus, hospital chaplaincy in Australia (and in most other Western countries) exists within a theoretical perspective that tends not to value its ministry and leads to "downsizing."

In light of this narrow economic approach, this article seeks to reflect critically upon hospital chaplaincy and the economic benefits that such a service already brings to health care institutions. While it is not possible to cover all the dynamics of economic rationalism and hospital chaplaincy, we raise the following core issues:

- economic rationalism and the hospital system,
- the value of hospital chaplaincy,
- economic downsizing,
- the chaplain's perspective of cost efficiency, and
- the challenge for hospital chaplaincy in the future.

We suggest that our Australian perspective contains lessons for other Western countries such as the United Kingdom, the United States of America, Canada and New Zealand who have a similar economic orientation among health policy makers.

1. ECONOMIC RATIONALISM

The term "economic rationalism" is used in a variety of contexts. In general terms one can define it as, "the goal of bringing the limited resources of society into proper relation with desired ends"[1] so as to achieve economic efficiency. At the broad level of social and health policy, economic rationalism during the latter part of the twentieth century may achieve needed gains in efficiency in terms of state action, and especially in terms of downsizing the bureaucracy. Yet, problems emerge when economic rationalism, via a market economy, espouses its own values that are uncritically assumed to be neutral and inherently good.

A critical understanding of the social construction of reality and the inherent embedded nature of values suggests that the market economy is not objective or value neutral but is a product of particular values that predominantly benefit the status quo. This can have numerous negative effects upon health care and chaplaincy. Such a system eschews communitarian and more wholistic notions of health care that are prized by many Australians who have attempted over the years to inform and reform their medical system. Secondly and ironically, in the name of the market, excessively large salaries and sums are paid to powerful players such as specialists; yet, the system fails to deliver adequate resources to those on welfare or with disabilities. Also, within such a system, those who are already powerful and have the resources, win; those who do not, lose. Pertinent questions consequently arise, "Whose knowledge counts?" and "What counts as costs and benefits?"

The social economist Pusey states that the inherent problem with market driven economic rationalism is, " . . . the loss of social intelligence given the number and range of potentially constructive discourses that have (consequently) been suppressed."[2] We believe that the philosophy of clinical pastoral care has been suppressed or rejected as inappropriate knowledge because it tends to be wholistic, egalitarian and concerned more for individual development than with institutional efficiency.

2. THE VALUE OF HOSPITAL CHAPLAINCY

The values and perspectives of hospital chaplains stand in stark contrast to current economic rationalism. A review of literature on the work of hospital chaplains indicates that their role, for example, is to "walk with people through the valley of anguish, denial, grief, loss, depression, anger and guilt, to stand at their side in the struggle with confusions and doubts, offer them love, hope and faith, and to work with them towards a realistic acceptance and accommodation of what the future will hold. . . ."[3] This process of chaplaincy ministry is what Mol[4] termed the sacralization (or re-sacralization) of one's identity. Based on that observation, Carey has noted that chaplains can help persons consolidate and stabilize in times of crisis or to encourage change/conflict when there is need for progression.[5]

However, what value does such ministry have in a market driven, or at least market influenced, public health care system? It could be argued that chaplaincy observed from an outside perspective might be viewed to be inherently inefficient. Yet, a chaplain deals with those things that the market mentality does not recognize as being important. What price do we give grief support, and what price the sacralization of identity and the support of people in their health care journey when these personal dynamics are not regarded as an important part of casemix funding?

The lack of support for Australian chaplaincy has often been couched in terms of "religiousness" and the importance of state and religion being separate since the Australian *Church and State Separation Act* of 1836. Yet, at another level it is worth asking, "But who else supports people in a holistic way in the spiritual aspects of their lives in the Australian health care system?" This is an especially important consideration when few other health professionals have the time to help patients with their essential emotional and spiritual journey. After all, it doesn't fit nicely into a funding formula.

Australian Chaplaincy Utility Research (AUS.CUR)

Despite this reality, or perhaps because of it, research in Australia has indicated that the majority of clinical staff tends to be highly favorable in their attitude towards the work of hospital chaplains. The Australian Chaplain Utility Research (AUS.CUR 1992-1995)[6] was developed and modified for the Australian scene (and in particular for the Royal Children's Hospital, Melbourne) from the North American 'Pastoral Care Survey' (NAPC 1972).[7] A significant development in the AUS.CUR survey was the inclusion of not only nurses and doctors but also all allied health personnel (e.g., physical therapists, speech pathologists, occupational therapists, audiologists, social workers, psychologists, musical therapists, play therapists, etc.). Some 390 clinical staff participated in the research.[8]

The research results were surprising, given the effects of secularization, modernization, professionalization and marginalization upon organized religion and its representatives in Australia. The AUS.CUR project clearly indicated that, while there was some criticism of hospital chaplains by clinical staff,[9] the majority of respondents (60%) and informants (88.2%) believed it was of "great importance" to have a chaplain's contribution as part of the hospital service. This was found to be true irrespective of staff gender, marital status, religious preference, years of service or professional specialization. Those working in intensive care and neonatal units expressed the most appreciation for chaplaincy; they frequently called on chaplains to assist staff and families during crises.

The major reasons given by staff interviewees for having resident chaplains within their working environment consisted of the following:

- teamwork (improving staff time management),
- providing religious and psycho-social support to patients and staff through such mechanisms as ritual, commitment religious literature, God, faith and the church,
- providing specialist support to families and staff particularly at times of death and grieving, and
- chaplain in-put into the hospital environment in terms of

  - bio-medical ethics,[10]
  - being a community link,
  - providing a non-diagnostic communication role within the hospital, and
  - alleviating emotional discomfort for staff and patients within a complex and sometimes frightening institution.[11]

Australian Liver Transplant and Hospital Chaplaincy Research

Preliminary results from more recent Australian research examined the role of chaplains in liver transplant units within three states (Victoria, Queensland and New South Wales). The Liver Transplant Unit and Hospital Chaplaincy research[12] suggests that a chaplain employed specifically by a transplant unit to care for patients and staff (i.e., The Austin Hospital, Melbourne) is highly appreciated. Unit staff members find them valuable in decision making (89%), assessing a patient's suitability for a transplant (89%), and providing personal assistance to staff (67%). Chaplains were also considered a help to the overall running of the unit (100%).

Of particular interest to policy makers and economic rationalists is that the research results gained from the three hospitals (averaged over years 1990-1994) also indicate "that the patients are being discharged at a faster rate than otherwise"[13] where a hospital chaplain is continually listening and drawing patients, relatives and staff members together to resolve issues. Though the research is not yet complete this is a very significant consideration when one considers the daily medical costs of transplants.

Indeed researchers, such as Homer and Hamilton[14] asserted that, through patient and staff support, chaplains can assist in reducing the need for drugs, emergency intervention or extended care, and thus play an important role in reducing overall medical costs. They suggested four main ways that the chaplains can help achieve these goals; they (i) provide spiritual counseling to facilitate treatment decisions; (ii) develop coping strategies for patients with illness/disabilities to facilitate treatment and discharge; (iii) provide emergency intervention for patients, and (iv) facilitate patient discharge to other organizations which provide adequate resources.

Australian 'Religious Volunteers'

Another issue that must be considered in terms of the economic value of hospital chaplaincy is the support services that hospital chaplains co-ordinate in terms of religious volunteers. While it is commonly known in Australia that the largest providers of non-government health and welfare services are the institutional churches, economists easily overlook the significant contribution of religious volunteers provided by churches to public institutions such as hospitals. Religious volunteers for example make up the fourth largest category of all Australian volunteers (17.7%), coming after Sport/Hobby (31.4%), Welfare/Community Volunteers (29.7%) and Education Volunteers (25.3%). Religious Volunteer numbers are more substantial than other volunteer categories such as, Emergency Services (4.9%), Arts/Culture (4.1%), Environment/animal welfare (3.7%), Business/Professional or union concerns (3.3%) or Law/Justice and political issues (1.7%). Indeed, it is a common view within church circles that religious volunteers regularly bolster the numbers of most other volunteer groups by giving a "helping hand" but seldom is assistance reciprocated to assist religious volunteers.[15]

It is also important to note, as described in Table 1, that religious volunteers each give among the highest percentage of hours in service per annum (> 300 hrs = 12%) totaling some 70 million hours of service. Religious volunteers give the longest period of service to the Australian community (> 10 years = 44.3%) with health and community welfare as one of their main fields of volunteer work (18%).

Hospital Chaplaincy Funding

The actual funding of Chaplains must also be considered, that is, "Who actually pays for the services of chaplaincy personnel?" In terms of cost for service, we argue that chaplaincy in Australia is very

TABLE 1. Australian Volunteers

	Religious Volunteers	Other Volunteers (High Category)*	Other Volunteers (Low Category)**
Field of Volunteering:	Religious 17.7%	Sport/Hobby 31.4%	Law/Politics 1.7%
Total Volunteer Hours Worked:	Religious 70.6m***	Sport/Hobby 105m	Foreign 2.7m
Volunteers > 300 Hrs:	Religious 12.0 %	Art/Culture 12.2%	Education 5.2%
Volunteering Time > 10yrs+:	Religious 44.3 %	Emergency 36.0%	Environment 14.0%
Health & Community Services:	Religious 18.0%	Welfare 29.2%	Art/Culture 2.0%

Notes: Data from: Australian Bureau of Statistics 'Voluntary Work' June 1995.

  *'Other volunteers' (High Category) = Highest Category of Volunteer contribution.
  **'Other volunteers' (Low Category) = Lowest Category of Volunteer Contribution.
  ***m = million hours.

cost efficient. The Australian Bio-Medical and Clinical Decision Making Research[16] involving over 300 part time and full time chaplaincy personnel (all members of the Australian Health and Welfare Chaplains Association), made clear that over 68% of hospital chaplaincy personnel are not remunerated from hospital budgets. These chaplains are reliant on church funding (40.3%) or self-funding (28.1%). Approximately 7% of chaplains receive mixed funding (from both church and hospital budgets). Only 24.1% of Australian chaplains are paid purely from hospital budgets. To put it bluntly–this means that a majority of hospitals are receiving a service with someone else footing the bill! (Figure 1).

3. DOWNSIZING OF HOSPITAL CHAPLAINCY

As yet there has been no research to assess the effects of 'devaluing' or 'downsizing' of hospital chaplaincy in Australia. The U.S. research reported later in this volume collates information from 370 chaplaincy department directors and is very timely. The results suggest that a significant number of U.S. departments have experienced budget cutbacks (27%).

FIGURE 1. Percentage of Australian Chaplaincy Personnel by Source of Remuneration

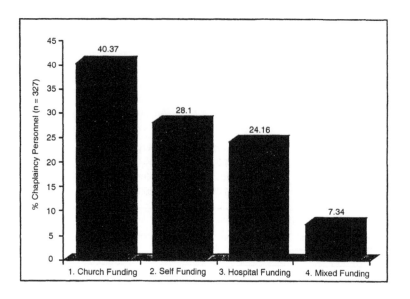

However, this same research notes that 45 percent have not experienced any budgetary differences up to the present time. Perhaps of some surprise is the result that 17 percent actually experienced growth in the department during this era of institutional downsizing (i.e., increased budget, staffing, etc.)? Further analysis revealed that larger departments more frequently experienced both more growth (24 vs. 39 departments) and budget cuts (35 vs. 60 departments) while smaller departments frequently reported that institutional down-sizing did not affect their budgets (49 vs. 37 departments) but more productivity was expected (46 vs. 32 departments).

While the authors note that these contradictory results regarding growth and downsizing suggest influential variable(s) beyond the scope of the research, some of these influential variables, in light of the AUS.CUR study, may be identifiable and provide understandable clues for the necessary adjustment and development of hospital chaplaincy ministry.

It may well be, of course, that these diverse results indicate that hospitals used different criteria as they cut staff positions. Some may have downsized all departments by an equal percentage. Other hospitals may have chosen to bring about some equality among departments, which would have necessitated a decrease in some departments but an increase in others. Indeed some smaller chaplaincy departments probably could not be downsized because it would mean their extinction. There are a host of possible reasons that make it difficult to speculate. Only further research, particularly qualitative studies, can provide further insight. Additionally, ideological considerations are important although they lie beyond economic and statistical approaches.

The AUS.CUR research sought to uncover these ideological considerations by including qualitative in-depth interviews in addition to its formal survey questionnaire. These interviews revealed numerous concerns from interdisciplinary staff regarding chaplains that would likely affect their downsizing or upsizing (as the case may be). Most of the comments were linked to the quality of chaplaincy ministry being performed and the mindset of key clinical staff and administrators responsible for making institutional decisions in regard to hospital chaplaincy.

The AUS.CUR results suggested that chaplains needed to increase their profile. Suggestions included poster displays, newsletters, brochures, increased visiting and training sessions for staff, each of which would be particularly informative in terms of the utility of chaplains beyond the more stereo-typical traditional roles of clergy. Second, in terms of teamwork, there was an obvious need to explore more productive ways in which teamwork can be enhanced among "competing" occupations within the hospital (e.g., between chaplains, social workers and psychologists), particularly where professional overlap exists in the delivery of psycho-social services for patients and their families. Several staff also noted the need for the pastoral care department to have a senior chaplain responsible for the internal teamwork management and oversight of other chaplains.

Third, chaplains need to be involved to a greater extent in ethics through, (i) their input on the hospital ethics committee, (ii) involvement in ethical decision making on the wards, (iii) at staff meetings and (iv) in the teaching or conducting of a regular ethics forum for the benefit of staff. Fourth in terms of personality and professional conduct, chaplains need to be, (i) good at social interaction, not shy but deliberate, friendly, smiling, chatty and up front about things,

(ii) flexible, not rigid in style or denominational traditionalism or belief but ecumenical and compassionate, and (iii) broad-minded with the capacity to listen.

Chaplains will likely appreciate the fifth result. Staff recognized that an increased number of chaplains are necessary if they are to successfully carry out their work in assisting patients, their families and staff. In light of the issues surrounding professional demarcation and current financial cutbacks, it is quite extraordinary to find that this was suggested by members from occupational groups other than chaplains. Indeed, the majority of interview respondents were strongly in favor of chaplaincy continuing. As stated by one allied health staff member: " . . . even though technology is so far advanced . . . , there are still people with feelings and I think that technology has created lots of other problems . . . I think that chaplains will be needed . . . well, people still have the same needs whether technology is here or not . . . " (AH 8).

Such recommendations, however, could be considered highly idiosyncratic, depending upon the institution and the chaplains. Herein, it can be argued, lies at least one answer to the variety of the US Downsizing survey results reported in this work. Chaplaincy departments, like the hospitals in which they reside, are intrinsically unique. Some chaplaincy departments and chaplains are highly proactive in their profile development, in their teamwork, in their involvement in ethical issues and ethical decision-making and are exemplary in their personal and professional pastoral conduct. Other chaplaincy departments and chaplains need improvement. It could be argued that those chaplaincy departments well developed in those areas noted above have developed a significant status, beyond the statistical records of pastoral output which have, in turn, led to up-grading.

Interestingly, the results of the US chaplaincy downsizing research gathered data concerning excellent strategic approaches for improving hospital chaplaincy not too dissimilar in thrust to that of the AUS.CUR study. These included increased communication with decision makers, greater teamwork by calling on powerful non-administrative personnel and increasing interdisciplinary involvements, developing relationship profile by building community support among institutional decision makers, develop research, and taking more responsibility for additional activities.

4. COST EFFICIENCY:
A HOSPITAL CHAPLAINCY PERSPECTIVE

Hospital administrators, health economists, and health policy advisers can achieve numerous advantages from the services of hospital chaplains. Some of these have already been suggested and the chaplains themselves confirm that. The BIO-MECDEM[17] research results mentioned earlier currently being conducted in Australia (and New Zealand[18]) provide comments from in-depth interviews concerning whether chaplains would consider hospital chaplaincy "a cost efficient service." The research, to be completed in 2000 AD, can currently be summarized as follows:

(i) Professional Service at a Reduced Fee Structure

Highly trained professional chaplains often receive salaries that no other professional grouping would tolerate, or indeed be allowed to tolerate. As one chaplain argues:

> I think for something like $30,000 (AU) a year, this hospital pays for a 24-hour-a-day-on-call service–I don't know another field of expertise where they can provide that sort of service for that relatively small of amount of money. [Hospital Chaplain 1]

Another chaplain suggests, as already noted above, that the services provided are largely paid for by sources outside of the health system:

> The [part time] hospital chaplaincy here is funded through a grant from local government and the churches around town prop that up by about $10-12,000 (AU) per year. So this hospital effectively gets an absolutely free service. [Hospital Chaplain 2]

Another chaplain suggests that chaplaincy can amount to exploitation:

> I get paid $13,000 a year . . . [by my parish] for my six days a week with a month's holiday and a week's retreat. So, I think it is quite unjust, to be perfectly honest. . . . I think the hospital takes advantage [of this]. The hospital where I am working is really supportive of chaplaincy but I think that if they had to front up to the actual cost of it, the financial cost of it, I think there would be some cutting back probably . . . I am not sure that they *couldn't*

afford it but I have a feeling that they *wouldn't* afford it. [Hospital Chaplain 3]

(ii) Patient and Staff Therapeutic Benefit

A chaplain who was a hospital patient relates the experience of receiving pastoral care and the importance of intangibles such as "love" and "healing":

> After having had pastoral care from a chaplain . . . I think that I'd rather be a patient receiving pastoral care from a chaplain than not. You go away with issues unresolved if you haven't had pastoral care from a chaplain. If you have, you can go away with the feeling that some one cares about you–somebody having shown love to you and that is an important part of your healing. [Hospital Chaplain 4]

We asked, "So how does that actually help the financial side of the hospital?" This patient/chaplain responded, "Well maybe the patient might not come back because they have been fully healed, and their families too, not just the patient" [Hospital Chaplain 4].

Another Australian chaplain points to the under-valued dimensions of chaplaincy, that which the accountants do not count:

> We are cost efficient. . . . because chaplains deal with so much grief that I believe we can help people to an extent that they may not have a result from their grief that will be physical. . . . Also . . . in bringing forth people's spirituality–it's there–but helping them to be aware of their spirituality that makes them whole somehow has an affect on their health. And it can have an affect on a relative's health too. [Hospital Chaplain 5]

Of course, here we face the problem of the lack of health research data regarding spirituality and the spiritual components of health. For many chaplains the effect is obvious, even though not included in economic modeling:

> Well, just that because people can get their anger out, I mean how often do chaplains go to see a patient and they tell you the next thing that 'bloody' happened wrong, you know and to help them talk it through–because chaplains are outside the system and the patient is not going to tell the doctor and the nurse that because

they'll get 'offside' but they will tell the chaplain–which can divert complications . . . when it [telling the chaplain] does happen I believe that it's helping them get well quicker. [Hospital Chaplain 6]

There are also other roles attested to by chaplains in the face of minimal hospital stays associated with the introduction of casemix in Australian hospitals:

> . . . with this whole crazy system . . . people coming into hospital for minimum lengths of time, invariably they're going out of hospital still with a great deal of pain or discomfort or the effects of their illness unresolved and if that is not worked through, then they can come back in a far worse state and it's actually not being efficient. You might as well have kept them in for an extra day than have them back in for a week. But if a chaplain can be there they can often discern the help that a patient might need to alert staff and prevent that. [Hospital Chaplain 7]

Another chaplain commented on a truly unique contribution although it is seldom discussed. Chaplains can give permission to terminal patients to die:

> Sometimes, though this sounds awful, sometimes we help people to let go and die quicker and so that's cost effective too. Or help the relatives let go. And I'm serious about that. [Hospital Chaplain 8]

(iii) Free Support Service

There is also the significant free service provided by lay and ordained pastoral volunteers. Few other trained persons who have valued roles would likely offer this free of charge. Love of service is something not easily valued in terms of neo-classical economics:

> Personally I come in here for free. I do it for nothing. . . . I do it for the love of the Lord. I am a Christian person and this (lay chaplaincy) is the way that I believe we should look after our sick people. [Volunteer Chaplain 1]

(iv) Additional Service

Another chaplain attests to the other ways in which a hospital may value a chaplain beyond economic recognition:

> I guess I gauge the seriousness of the hospital by the comments that come to me and by the way that the chaplain is part of the emergency procedures of the hospital, just like a specialist is paged, like other emergency staff, so is the chaplain–so we do more than traditional stuff! [Hospital Chaplain 10]

There are also other ways that chaplains help, even though these may not be included in any formal regime. As one chaplain suggests:

> A chaplain can often discern the help that a patient might need, and put them in touch with resources that will be there for them in the community. Um, and I'm not just talking about community based nursing care . . . so there's a whole heap of little things that mean the patient's stay will be far more comfortable and the patient themselves will be better cared for because of all the little things that a chaplain does. [Hospital Chaplain 11]

Likewise, extensive pastoral care associated with death and dying is hardly recompensed by funeral fees, and pastoral care can be ongoing:

> For the social worker, the viewing and funeral is the end of the process but for chaplain it can be ongoing . . . So, in a sense then, through the chaplain, the hospital, in a way, has an ongoing pastoral link and also promotional link with the family in terms of a positive outcome about their hospital experience. If there is another hiccup in the family or somebody else is sick or something else happening they will come back to the chaplain and seek further assistance because there has been a relationship established there. [Hospital Chaplain 12]

5. THE CHALLENGE FOR CHAPLAINCY

While one can argue that hospitals and health systems do not value the full worth of hospital chaplaincy, chaplains themselves do not seem to fully value their own worth.

> I don't think chaplains value themselves enough–value their worth–because they tend to say, 'Oh, I'll do it because I am a Christian,' or 'I'll do it because that is what God expects me to do.' I don't agree with that at all. [Hospital Chaplain 13]

This stark statement reveals much. In particular, the secular world within which chaplains minister provides little systemic affirmation to them. All other professionals are paid more and, in a largely secular Australian society, being Christian or doing "God's business" is not highly esteemed. Chaplains contribute to this problem by the lack of highly credentialed professionals and the lack of research results in the field. Experienced chaplains, and those with CPE background, know the importance of their ministry, but they conduct little economically relevant research regarding their contribution. Likewise, research is needed as regards the effectiveness of chaplaincy, not just in terms of neo-classical economics reified into economic rationalism, but in terms of the totality of the disputed socio-political space which is "care."

In conclusion, economic rationalism constitutes a significant force in Australian health care and chaplains have not sufficiently researched their cost efficiency. Qualitative research suggests that chaplains stand for values that are not incorporated into the economic rationalist formula. These values may constitute "rejected knowledge" that does not fit into the system; thus it is not recognized and counted.[19] It seems clear that in Australian hospitals, chaplaincy is seen as the bargain basement special, often highly valued by individuals, but seldom incorporated into the economic rationalist formula of modern health systems. The U.S. research reported here highlights some important aspects in terms of strategies to be employed in the future if chaplaincy wishes to remain beyond the next century. The challenge now is to build upon the insights of the quantitative and qualitative research found here and elsewhere.

NOTES

1. Michan, E.J. (1985). "Economic efficiency." In: Kuper, A. and Kuper, J., *Social Science Encyclopedia*, London: Routledge & Kegan Paul, p. 226.

2. *Ibid.,* p. 22

3. Carey, L.B. (1991). "Clergy under the knife: A review of literature on hospital chaplains." *Ministry Journal of Continuing Education*, Sydney, Summer, p. 7-9.

4. Mol, H. (1976/77). *Identity and the sacred: A sketch for a new social scientific theory of religion*. Oxford: Blackwell, p. 5.

5. Carey, L.B. (1998). "The sacralization of identity: A cross-cultural and interreligious paradigm for hospital chaplaincy." *Journal of Health Care Chaplaincy*, Cambridge, p. 15-24.

6. Carey, L.B. (1995). "The utility of hospital chaplains in health care institutions: A case study of the Royal Children's Hospital (Melbourne, Australia)." Unpublished Research, Behavioral Health Sciences, La Trobe University, Victoria, Australia.

7. Carey, R. (1972). "Hospital chaplains: Who needs them?" *The Catholic Hospital Association*, St. Louis, Missouri, USA.

8. Carey, L.B., Aroni, R., Edwards, A. (1997). "Health policy and well being: Hospital chaplaincy." In: Gardner, H., *Health Policy in Australia*, Oxford University Press, Melbourne, p. 190-210.

9. The criticisms/suggestions are discussed later in this paper.

10. Carey, L.B., Aroni, R.A., Edwards, A. (1996). "Medical ethics and the role of hospital chaplains." *Ministry, Society & Theology* (Melbourne), 10, 2, p. 66-79.

11. Carey, L.B. (1997). "The role of hospital chaplains: A research overview." *Journal of Health Care Chaplaincy*, Cambridge, p. 3-11.

12. Elliot, H. (1996). "Liver transplant units and hospital chaplaincy." Ph.D. Research, Religious Studies Department, Sydney University.

13. Elliot, H. & Carey, L.B. (1996). "The hospital chaplain's role in an organ transplant unit." *Ministry, Society & Theology*, Melbourne, Vol.10, No. 1, p. 66-78.

14. Homer, L.C. & Hamilton, M.A. (1984). "Pastoral care: Social services role in reducing medical costs." *Hospital Progress*, Vol. 65, No. 6, pp. 50-62.

15. Trewin, D. (1996). "Voluntary work, Australia," Australian Bureau of Statistics, Commonwealth of Australia, Catalogue No. 4441.0.

16. Carey, L.B. (1996-2000). *BIO-MECDEM: Bio-Medical Ethics and Clinical Decision Making and the Role of Hospital Chaplains in Australia and New Zealand.* School of Public Health, La Trobe University, Victoria, Australia.

17. *Ibid.*, Carey, L.B. (1996-2000).

18. Carey, L.B., Aroni, R., Gronlund, M. (1998). "Biomedical ethics, clinical decision making and hospital chaplaincy in New Zealand." *Ministry, Society & Theology* (Melbourne), Vol. 12, No. 2, p. 136-156.

19. Newell, C. 1994. "The Social Construction of the Wheelchair and the Cochlear Implant: A Study of the Definition and Regulation of Disability." Unpublished Ph.D. thesis, School of Social Inquiry, Deakin University, Geelong, Victoria.

The Moon Has Four Phases
and That's What Worries Me

Art Lucas, MDiv

SUMMARY. The values held by health care administrators and inherent in the operation of the institution are of primary importance to the ministry of pastoral care. This narrative/story provides a case history in which the author recounts how these values change as administrators change. The results suggest that these values constitute one of the hidden variables that influenced the questionnaire results reported earlier in this work. *[Article copies available for a fee from The Haworth Document Delivery Service: 1-800-342-9678. E-mail address: <getinfo@haworthpress inc.com> Website: <http://www.haworthpressinc.com>]*

KEYWORDS. Clergy, chaplain, pastoral counseling, pastoral care, health care reform

My nine years as Director of Spiritual Care are marked by three distinct funding phases. In the first phase, Department funding came when we demonstrated contributions to the institution's clinical processes. The second reflected firm executive support for contributions to the health of the communities we served. The third consisted of demands for cost reduction while emphasizing compassionate care. In all but the third, the department has thrived, developed and grown.

Even in the best of times, professionals in other disciplines sought more services from us than we could provide. This was related, at least

Art Lucas is affiliated with The Department of Spiritual Care, Barnes-Jewish Hospital, Washington University Medical Center, 1 Barnes Jewish Hospital Plaza, St. Louis, MO 63110-1094.

[Haworth co-indexing entry note]: "The Moon Has Four Phases and That's What Worries Me." Lucas, Art. Co-published simultaneously in *Journal of Health Care Chaplaincy* (The Haworth Pastoral Press, an imprint of The Haworth Press, Inc.) Vol. 10, No. 1, 2000, pp. 53-67; and: *Professional Chaplaincy: What Is Happening to It During Health Care Reform?* (ed: Larry VandeCreek) The Haworth Pastoral Press, an imprint of The Haworth Press, Inc., 2000, pp. 53-67. Single or multiple copies of this article are available for a fee from The Haworth Document Delivery Service [1-800-342-9678, 9:00 a.m. - 5:00 p.m. (EST). E-mail address: getinfo@haworthpressinc.com].

in part, to our continuous development in one clinical area or another. Adequate response to needs was difficult when our own boundaries were moving. Additionally, as Department Director, I always wanted a clear multidisciplinary picture of the necessity of any additional pastoral staffing and was careful about adding the most appropriate level of staffing in terms of required professional skills, clinical integration, and continuity of care. More than once when we have experienced an across the board budget cut at the hospital, I have kicked myself for not building in "fat" that I could trim before getting to what we really needed in order to provide essential care. In the material below, I describe the context and characteristics of each phase and then draw some conclusions that seem evident to me concerning the relentless pressure of cost containment.

PHASE ONE: CLINICAL CONTRIBUTIONS

When I arrived at the hospital in 1990, Administration wanted its long-standing pastoral care department to become more involved in multidisciplinary teams. The Department had a long history that included participation in the St. Louis Cluster of the Association for Clinical Pastoral Education (ACPE) with a clinical pastoral education (CPE) program. The Department was mostly organized along denominational lines; Catholic priests visited Catholic patients, CPE residents and interns visited all others on their assigned floors. One staff chaplain was assigned to the Lung Transplant program and a few other floors. The administrative and clinical leadership valued the pastoral care service they had and vaguely knew they wanted something more that increased participation in clinical areas, something more integrated with the clinical emphasis of the hospital.

We began with rebuilding our Pastoral Care Advisory Committee to oversee the Department and its CPE program. We included administrators, physicians, nurses, social workers, middle managers, and community clergy in the review process. We interviewed clinical leadership at all levels, including the medical chiefs of all the Washington University School of Medicine services, the nursing administrator associated with each of those services, the head nurse for each patient care unit, and the leading physician for each unit. Rather than ask what they wanted from pastoral care, we asked each to tell us about his/her vision for the service/unit during the next five or ten years. We thought it was inappropriate to ask them what they wanted from pastoral care because that would expect them to be the experts. That was our role. Asking for their vision engaged them on a level of values and direction, a level on which we could join them in dialogue.

That set the stage for our development in Phase One. Concern was already rising about decreasing remuneration due to the rapidly rising managed care penetration around the country, a little more slowly in St. Louis. HMOs and PPOs and all the other alphabet soup of market place solutions for the socially defined problem of rising health care costs were cutting into the financial margins of the hospital and therefore into the funds they believed they could use for growth or development. By the time we had developed a mission statement and strategic plan, the hospital was experiencing a tight budget and making occasional cuts. Administration, even given their strong affirmation of care for the religious/spiritual dimension of our patients, families and staff, needed a clear, substantive reason to spend any new money. All our plans, however, were eventually approved.

We adopted a new organization for our staff and services around clinical areas. We tracked patient experiences from admissions, through clinical interventions, through transfers among floors, to discharge and into outpatient, follow up care at the hospital. These tracks became sets of assignments, still using nursing/patient care units as the building blocks. Each chaplain, including CPE students, became the "Anchor Chaplain" for one or more tracks. S/he was to anchor the pastoral care for the patients, families and staff of the track, not provide all that was needed, but anchor it. The chaplain who was part of the Lung Transplant service became the Anchor Chaplain for Thoracic Tracks. A chaplain resident became the Anchor Chaplain for the Heart Tracks. In later developments, the hospital adopted a clinical service line (CSL) approach and we were ready. Our tracks did not exactly match what eventually became the CSLs, but we were close and we were accustomed to the perspective.

We approached proposals for additional staffing as a request from the clinical area. As Director of Pastoral Care, I was the expert consultant to the clinical leadership in defining the staffing resource most appropriate to the current clinical needs. Regardless of how the discussions were initiated, the next step was to talk with clinicians in the area about the clinical picture. We were particularly interested in identifying any changes in the area's population that might shed light on the changed utilization of chaplaincy. We would revisit the original vision for the clinical service and our pattern of providing pastoral care to it.

Once we identified what chaplaincy could contribute to the care of the patients and the development of the clinical service, I took on the task of recommending what staffing was best. I would consider/reconsider our key staffing values of skills, integration, continuity to determine the appropriate level of additional staffing, i.e., volunteers, contract community clergy, CPE Externs/Interns, CPE resident, CPE second year resident, anchor chaplain. How many hours a week were needed? If more than one full-time person were needed to meet needs and expectations, I would always propose only the first staffing increment. The intention was always to stay responsibly conservative, start with one addition and let experience tell us what is next.

I would consider other clinical areas that were utilizing chaplaincy to see if any partial staffing could be reasonably put together with some other needs to make a better whole staffing solution. If that were the case, I would talk with the clinical leadership in that second area about their patients and clinical strategic plans. For instance, a second year CPE resident might bring the requisite level of skills and ability to a given area, but the pool of interested CPE applicants might not be sufficiently steady to ensure that we could fill a position year after year. And, of course, placing a CPE student in a position assumed that it was a good context for learning.

I would then write up a proposal for the clinical leadership in the area(s), including a brief history of pastoral care in that area and current experience. The proposal would then describe projections about patient demographics, a sketch of their clinical experience, volume, acuity, changes (like new services about to be offered) and what a chaplain dedicated to the area(s) could contribute. The proposal would then sketch the staffing necessary to make those contributions, the rationale for that particular staffing (again in terms of skill, integration and continuity), what the staffing would cost, what we could expect and what indices would exist to let us know if the contributions were being made. We would talk though the ideas, make changes as needed and end up with a proposal for staffing on which we all agreed. Occasionally my initial ideas were far enough off to have to go through the whole proposal development cycle again.

The final proposal would then go to hospital administration with a cover memo from the key clinical leadership (at least the head nurse or nurse coordinator, medical chief or medical director) and myself, conveying the request for additional pastoral care staff. The request memo always had at least three names as the authors, sometimes more if a perspective from social work or employee assistance were important to the picture. I would present it to the Vice-President to whom I reported as a staffing/budget request for the clinical service regarding pastoral care. Our recommendations were very often approved, despite a policy of financial constraints.

Support for chaplaincy in Phase One had two bases. The first was the basic positive regard the hospital administration had for pastoral care as part of what a hospital should make available to patients, families and staff. All we needed to do was actively appreciate their respect of us, be cognizant of the values their regard reflected, and keep them informed/involved in the life of the Department. This was generally true throughout the hospital although there were exceptions. Some leadership in the finance area always seemed to have difficulty grasping pastoral care as anything more than a socially appropriate nicety that should be provided by the churches. Pastoral care, at best, was on the fringe and expendable if resource problems existed.

The second was the administrator's and clinician's prime values, including:

- the development of clinical service for patients and families (the hospital truly saw itself, as our motto on the history wall said, "leading healthcare into the 21st century"), and
- a view of the patient as a person rather than a disease process or body part.

The distribution of increasingly tight resources was governed by asking what it would take to give "premier" or "gold standard" care for patients and families as well as what it would take to lead healthcare. The job of the Pastoral Care Director was to make it as easy as possible for the hospital leadership to make the right decision about pastoral care staffing by tying our requests to the values that were held as the most important for the future of the hospital. We were always about meeting people where they were, especially in terms of beliefs/ values, and we applied that to the people who led the Hospital as well as patients, family members, and staff. Clear, crisp, focused recommendations in terms of service and the whole person were essential.

The dialogue was always within the hospital structures, caregivers and leaders, never extending to the hospital Board of Trustees. Leaving the Trustees out of the dialogue was a mistake. I suspected so at the time and am sure in retrospect. The Trustees' vision of the hospital was increasingly important as strategic decisions concerning its business viability drew closer and closer every day.

PHASE TWO: SYSTEM SUPPORT
AND COMMUNITY FOCUS

In June, 1993 Barnes Hospital (including Barnes Hospital at Washington University Medical Center, Barnes Hospital West County, Barnes St. Peters Hospital, and Barnes Extended Care in Clayton), Jewish Hospital, and the Christian Health System (including Christian Hospital NE/NW, Alton [Illinois] Memorial Hospital, Boone Medical Center [Columbia, Mo.] and affiliated hospitals in southwest Illinois and southeast Missouri) merged to form Barnes-Jewish-Christian (BJC) Health System, with Fred Brown, F.A.C.H.E., as the President and Chief Executive Officer. A committed United Methodist layman and past president of the American Protestant Hospital Association, Mr. Brown had long been convinced of the importance of pastoral care in health care. Mr. Brown's primary screen for decision making was whether something was "the right thing to do." The shorthand version of the new BJC mission was to "Improve the health of the people and communities we serve." Within weeks of the formation of BJC, Mr. Brown called together the leaders of pastoral care from the entities within the System. We formed the BJC Spiritual Care Council (BJC SCC). Mr. Brown's charge to us went something like this:

> If BJC is to provide premier health care for the people in the communities we serve, we will need to have premier pastoral care as a part of what we do. I want you to get your brains out of your buildings, envision what premier pastoral care would be for the System and for the population we serve, develop a plan for that pastoral care, tell me what it will cost and what we can expect from it. When you have it together you will present it to the System Executive Council for approval. Any questions?

We were smart enough to say, "OK" and to ask no questions. We talked with him a bit more about his vision for BJC and excused ourselves to get down to work on a vision and plan.

After more time than we ever dreamed it would take and more

learning than we thought possible, we gave the plan to Mr. Brown for his review and then to the Executive Council for approval. It had been difficult and challenging work. The plan addressed staffing in the entities, community education, professional education (including and not limited to CPE), research, community based care, support for entity staff (including chaplains) and physicians, developing a pastoral care foundation, communication, and other aspects. Our strategic plan for pastoral care received Executive Council approval in the midst of a substantive conversation directly facilitated by Mr. Brown's clear leadership. He made it plain that a pastoral care plan, this one or another, would be an integral part of the System's overall strategic plan. Since the Executive Council included the Senior Executive Officer from each of the System's major entities (hospital, extended care facility, home health and hospice, community clinics, etc.), approval of the plan meant at least initial support for parts of the plan that had implications for a given entity. As the System continued to grow, so did the Spiritual Care Council, coming to include chaplains from three additional institutions that were brought into the system.

From that point on, the development of pastoral care within the system was related as an integral part to the BJC SCC strategic plan. The SCC would identify the next step of the plan to implement, work with the administration and leadership in the related area to refine the idea to be implemented, and request funding. When the steps to be implemented clearly benefited a given entity in the System, the first point for funding decisions was always the entity and its leadership. At BJH that often received a favorable response. There were a number of reasons for this support:

- the same generally positively disposed to pastoral care leadership was still largely in place,
- the staff or programmatic growth was consistently perceived as in line with BJH's strategic plan, an alignment I had worked to assure in my contributions to the SCC plan,
- BJH leadership saw itself as playing a visible, leading role in the previously competing entities that were now becoming a unified System, and
- BJH continued to have the resources to do what it truly saw as important.

The recommendations were generally presented in the format described above to which the leadership had become accustomed, with an added section, now, on how this increment was related to or an explicit part of the (previously approved) BJC SCC strategic plan for pastoral care. Each recommendation and the concomitant request for funding, staffing, space, and equipment was firmly contextualized in the bigger pictures of BJH's care for patients, families and staff as well as for the people in the communities we served. The cost/benefit picture was as clear as we could make it and included indices by which we would measure its contribution.

In other entities SCC colleagues had different experiences based on the different immediate values. Some moved fairly aggressively, others did not. At BJH we were aggressive with the same basic conservatism described above.

When we had steps to take in implementing the plan that would benefit more than one entity or for the benefits of which no entity could be clearly associated, the SCC went to Mr. Brown for approval and funding. For example, we envisioned an ACPE Certified Supervisor to roam the BJC service area (in eastern Missouri and southwestern Illinois) and offer community-based CPE. The idea was that we would offer training to community clergy because more health care was shifting to the communities, because pastoral care was an integral part of that care, and because these community resource persons would have to incorporate increasing responsibilities into their ministries. It was the right thing to do. For initiatives such as this, Mr. Brown created a separate budgetary cost center, placed within the BJH Spiritual Care budget structure for "System Spiritual Care Initiatives."

The SCC also developed an alternate approach for recommendations from the entity level for which there was universal affirmation and for which funding was not available. Representatives of the Council and leadership from the entity would write a request to Mr. Brown for System funding in the form of additional budget cap room in order to be able to implement the SCC plan based recommendation. This cap approach quickly turned into simply putting the budget for these items in the BJC Pastoral Care cost center. When these plans were approved a plan of descending support was put into place. For instance, to fund the additional one-half FTE required to initiate CPE programming at Barnes-Jewish St. Peters Hospital, BJC put in the full amount for Year 1, 75 percent for Year 2, 50 percent in Year 3, 25 percent in Year 4 and none in year five, expecting BJSPH to pick up the increasing difference progressively. Mr. Brown's reasoning was that he wanted to make it as easy as possible for the entity administrators to do the right thing without immediately feeling the full weight on their budgetary bottom lines in the midst of the growing budgetary pressure on everyone.

Mr. Brown reiterated his support for spiritual care throughout the System in each budget building season, noting the two departments that were not to be cut: spiritual care and internal audit. The pair reflected his way of holding together both his commitments to the heart of health care and his tough, accountable business sense. When someone in administration tested this, he quickly made it clear that his "do not touch" directive was serious. Not only did this provide effective, specific protection from across the board cuts at different entities, it also gave an extremely substantive message about the importance of pastoral care in his vision of BJC.

Believe it or not, there was a downside to all of this.

- Once again, as I had done in Phase One, the SCC for the System and I again for BJH, never effectively engaged the BJC *Board* or the BJH *Board* about spiritual care. Even though it was in our plan, we did not educate the boards throughout the System about pastoral care and its place within health care.
- Some leadership persons in the network quietly concluded that they did not need to provide budget support for spiritual care. Others quietly saw pastoral care as "Mr. Brown's thing" and thought no more about it.
- The SCC and its efforts consumed increasing amounts of the members' time and energy, not so much as our plans got bigger, but as the System became more than an aggregate of entities. Mr. Brown was leading a centralized vision with autonomous, accountable components. As more was approached as a system, like clergy notification, community clergy benefits, clinical service lines, community wellness programming, and partnering with congregations/business/schools, more was demanded to think, plan, implement, and evaluate as a system. Our attention was drawn away from the increasing tensions with more entity-focused concerns.
- Our relationship with Mr. Brown made it virtually impossible for the SCC to look to the day, whenever that day might be, when the top leadership of BJC would be in the hands of another person.

- While I am proud to say that the SCC never took advantage of the administrative support to fatten its larder toward lean times, we repeated the conservative approach from Phase One.

In summary, our development in Phase Two was based on:

- executive vision, strong approval, and high expectations of pastoral care as a necessary part of "premier health care," and
- the strong working consensus with which the BJC SCC was eventually able to work once we got our brains out of our buildings and fought real good.

PHASE THREE: "IT'S THE COSTS, DUMMY!"

In August of 1998, Mr. Brown stepped aside in order to give his full attention to his upcoming tenure as the Chairman of the American Hospital Association. At the same time, new leadership of the BJC Board was coming into power and this new Board both named an Interim COE and began a national search. All this was occurring just as the first shadows were appearing from the awesome negative financial impact of the Balanced Budget Act of 1997. The new leadership was committed to attacking fiscal issues it felt had received too little attention or secondary priority by the first generation of BJC leadership. The Interim CEO was committed to immediately reducing System costs in order to brace for the onslaught of effects from the Balanced Budget Act.

All those changes combined for a change of corporate values more sweeping than I would have dreamed possible. Those in the entities, at the administrative and board levels, who had never liked the centralized direction of BJC, welcomed these changes and soon BJC was more like an affiliation of entities than a unified system. Soon all the emphases on the communities disappeared and were replaced by emphases on cost effective, then affordable, medical care.

I was personally deeply shaken. It seemed to me the vicissitudes of power and "what have you done for me lately" were about to turn a health care system into another business conglomerate. What so shook me was not so much the change in BJC although that would have been enough. What got to my bones was the seemingly facile radical break with a carefully built past, a past as recent as just yesterday was suddenly gone.

The driving value right now in BJC is the elimination of costs. The Act's crushing effects on teaching hospitals intensifies the pressure. This is the driver I had always feared. Few purchases, if any, are essential when cost is the driving force. That leaves pastoral care particularly vulnerable because it has always been a stranger in a strange land. Chaplaincy is in between health care providers as well as faith communities and only on the edge of their consciousness. We are non-essential to both of them, even with our best efforts at integration, at affirming the added clinical and customer satisfaction value of pastoral care. Even studies demonstrating the positive economic impact of professional pastoral care won't help. At worst we are expenses the religious communities should bear. To faith communities we are often praised, often valuable outgrowths broken off into the outside world of medicine and now business. At worst we are traitors who have sold out for pieces of silver. In that boundary life, as Dr. Peggy Way so profoundly described us during the recent Association of Professional Chaplains annual meeting in Kansas City, we are "in a pinch," on the margin, expendable.

Given almost any value, I have always been confident we could take responsibility for our substantive contribution to the care of people. If the value is cost reduction, we are just an expense. The only good news is: so is absolutely everyone else; doctor, nurse, administrator, accountant, phlebotomist, pharmacist, discharge coordinator, parking attendant, . . . all costs. The trouble is that this is a hard truth for any of us to incorporate. So those on the margin are identified more easily.

At BJH we have been treated fairly given the cost reduction process. BJH Spiritual Care Services has received the same across the board percentage cuts as all the other departments and services in our group. We are considered ancillary services along with virtually every other direct patient care service except physicians and nursing. The latter two are considered direct patient care and the budget cuts there are less. Cuts to support services such as accounting, billing office, and human resources are deeper. And as Director, I have the responsibility and flexibility of figuring out how to get those costs out. I have yet to be told to cut a specific existing position. I am able to talk long and hard both with my staff and with my vice-president about the trade-offs involved in any reduction. Because we have never been fully adequate to our mission, to others' growing expectations of us, because I never drove us to fatten up, every cut directly reduces our ability to provide the service for patients, families and staff. That means either someone else picks it up while they are being reduced too or it simply goes undone. When it goes undone something we incorporated as a considered component of quality care is gone.

Department directors or line chaplains out there who believe that evidence of efficacy buys security are deluding themselves. A secure place for professional chaplaincy in health care will not be created by professional developments in the field, by studies or positive research results. Given the current, over-riding value throughout health care attributed to cost reduction, nothing, *no one is secure.* We are *all* costs. Hospital administrators and leaders are increasingly aware that they cannot afford all they believe to be important for quality care. Attempts to demonstrate that pastoral care is important and essential does not secure anything except perhaps the increased personal pain of some administrators as our ability to give care reduces with, if not faster than, our costs.

Please be clear; my wrath is aimed at the society that decided to entrust the reduction of health care costs and access problems to the marketplace and the resultant commoditization of health care. The more society sees health care as an expense to the production of "real goods and services" (until one needs health care), the more any other value must fight for its existence. My dismay is at the speed with which BJC leadership feels forced to incorporate (pun intended) this value.

At the BJC level, the new era has reversed the previous pastoral care development modalities. As the System became more decentralization, our cost center budget has been dispersed the to entities that actually provided and benefited from the services. From a decentralizing perspective, it was the right thing to do because it supported the effected positions and programs. The leadership also went to great pains to make sure the process and outcome of the decentralization of the BJC PC cost center was budget neutral to everyone. They made sure it was not a soft way for BJH to look good in cutting costs nor a hard addition of costs only to the other entities. Even then, some of the entity administrators who had accepted pastoral care as a free bonus of the previous corporate era have cut the new positions. Others have stepped up and assumed the added expense. Still others have assumed the expense and become much more isolated in how they use or direct the service, believing the SCC to be a relic of an old centralized era.

At BJH, the new Senior Executive Officer has instituted a major emphasis on providing *compassionate* care for patients and families. Even with the clear identification of compassion as a key value, we have difficulty engaging it with our new leadership, *so far*. Compassion is such an assumed part of spiritual care that it is easily overlooked. And I still struggle with how to help our visibility on that screen. Other professionals are highlighted for their *acts* of compassion, and rightly so. Such acts, however, are every-day occurrences for chaplains who vivify and weave them through their clinically integrated care. Indeed, compassion is an important quality of care that can be improved throughout any clinical area and within every caregiver. This can be done independent of concerns about staffing, acuity levels, remuneration schemes. Its emphases are intra personal and relational–where the longest traditions of pastoral care have been for decades. All that combines for difficulty in applying compassion as a value in the BJH context for Spiritual Care Service development. Of course, we should and can focus on enriching compassion without regard to the resources we have or do not have, whatever care we can or cannot provide, whatever development or research we are or are not capable of pursuing. We are, however, finding it very difficult to engage this emphasis on cost cutting and focus on compassion because values, visions, and mission seem to mean something different now.

We are directed to fund-raising to meet development or even maintenance costs. While health care certainly needs all the outside funding it can garner, grants and gifts are not the sort of funding which can support core programming. It can be great for projects with a definable beginning-middle-end like research and pilot projects. It is not a healthy support for everyday staffing of services.

My development strategy for BJH Spiritual Care Services and that of the SCC for system pastoral care initiatives has moved to emphasize education, education of administration, middle management, and, finally, board members. At BJH we put together a 3-ring binder containing:

- a brief description of professional chaplaincy including the requirements for Board Certification in the specialty (a real shocker for many who have read it),
- a brief description of clinically integrated direct patient spiritual care including the clinical service line organization, integration and accountability,

- publications authored or co-authored by members of the department in professional journals (I guess I am still reaching for vestiges of the old Barnes value of leadership in health care.),
- articles written about us and published in hospital/system publications, the local press, and national publications such as that of the American Hospital Association,
- letters written to us by patients and family members expressing their appreciation for our care, choosing especially those which shed light beyond the religious practices and basic support functions of our care,
- letters written to us in evaluation/appreciation by those who have spent time at BJH to learn about how we go about giving pastoral care so they can transpose some back to their own setting, and
- articles providing a basic background for the place of faith, beliefs, values and religion in health care in general including foci in healing, wellness and patient satisfaction.

So far the response of those who have read it has been almost uniformly shock-to-surprise at what it takes to be a professional chaplain and at the complex and substantive discipline for pastoral care giving we have developed at BJH.

In the face of raw cost reductions and the sense that nothing else "really" matters, it is easy for me to feel fearful, fearful for my own future, fearful for the future of chaplains in the Department, and fearful for the future of what professional chaplains bring to the patients. I find it hard, however, to behave as if nothing else "really" matters. I know much more matters, including the presence, faithfulness, compassion, skill and the contribution professional chaplains uniquely bring. So I have to be faithful to them and assert our portion of the "much more" for those in leadership positions who must make the seemingly impossible, no-win decisions about where to expend our increasingly precious resources of money. And I have to make those assertions in whatever ways are easiest for the leadership to understand and incorporate while constantly holding the authenticity of the messages. I am left with being faithful. I suppose that is not a bad fall back position for somebody with my job description. And it is a very interesting constant mix of fear, rage, exhaustion, and importance.

From that position I can envision fresh *strategic planning* flowing out of these current developments. *Strategic thinking* seems to be a constant in the development we have been able to maintain to date, whatever some of the other variables may be. That is within my control. Another constant seems to be *leadership positively inclined for pastoral/spiritual care* or ultimately supportive of it. I do not believe I can control that. I can educate and I can *educate* those leaders, including board members I have failed to engage before. And another constant is the role of the culture's values, as distinct from those of an individual leader. I cannot control that. What I can do is the same that professional chaplains have always done, do my best to *meet those values whether and with whom they are* while maintaining my own faithfulness.

PHASE FOUR: THE MOON HAS FOUR PHASES AND THAT'S WHAT WORRIES ME. . . .

At this moment, the only option on which I am clear is to stay faithfully engaged!

OBSERVATIONS ON BOOKS, JOURNALS, AND ARTICLES RELEVANT TO PROFESSIONAL CHAPLAINCY AND HEALTH CARE REFORM

These comments reflect on the theme of this publication. Certainly much has been written, albeit not in book format, about the impact of downsizing, elimination of programs, and related concerns that are often the immediate crises created by reform.

The fascinating aspect of the challenge is to look beyond these symptoms! Such explorations are vitally important if we are to identify creative and appropriate responses to the challenges ahead. As Daniel F. Chambliss said in his book, *Beyond Caring* (University of Chicago Press, 1996):

> ... (the) problems transcend the individual motivations of actors; they instead reveal structural features of the setting. . . . They are problems not of persons but of the system. Thus, our tasks are both etiological as well as ontological. One does need to study the causes and reasons for the current crisis. One must also explore the very nature of the organism itself for possible causes.

Several years ago, Richard G. Cote suggested a similar view in his book, *Re-Visioning Mission: The Catholic Church & Culture in Postmodern America* (Paulist Press, 1996):

> It is a function of the Spirit, as Jews and Christians have known it, to enter searchingly into [one's] house, and there to put ques-

[Haworth co-indexing entry note]: "Observations on Books, Journals, and Articles Relevant to Professional Chaplaincy and Health Care Reform." Moyer, Frank S. Co-published simultaneously in *Journal of Health Care Chaplaincy* (The Haworth Pastoral Press, an imprint of The Haworth Press, Inc.) Vol. 10, No. 1, 2000, pp. 69-77; and: *Professional Chaplaincy: What Is Happening to It During Health Care Reform?* (ed: Larry VandeCreek) The Haworth Pastoral Press, an imprint of The Haworth Press, Inc., 2000, pp. 69-77. Single or multiple copies of this article are available for a fee from The Haworth Document Delivery Service [1-800-342-9678, 9:00 a.m. - 5:00 p.m. (EST). E-mail address: getinfo@haworthpressinc.com].

tions, now like a breath, now like a wind, to try all things that it finds there, to question their fitness to endure . . . It is a delusion to suppose that the disturbing questions will, if ignored, go away; if suppressed, be forgotten; or that by hiding ourselves like naked Adam we can escape them. It is no less delusive to expect that we shall get comforting answers to our questionings. To live with our uncertainties is not simply a necessary part of our education at all levels; it is the very truth of faith. To endure the sifting process of interrogation is the hallmark of discipleship.

It is interesting and hopeful that some signs of the present crisis, as well as possible steps for resolution, were identified by past leaders in our field. Below, I describe four contributions that cast unique light on current concerns.

1. Paul Tillich. "The Theology of Pastoral Care" *Proceedings of the Fifth National Conference on Clinical Pastoral Education.* The Advisory Committee on Clinical Pastoral Education 1958.

Dr. Tillich, in an address delivered November 9, 1956, spoke to at least one of the roots of today's malady.

When I hear the term pastoral care, I sometimes imagine myself to be in the situation of receiving pastoral care, and imagining this, I somehow feel humiliated. Someone else makes me an object of his care, but no one wants to become an object and, therefore, he resists such situations like pastoral care. Is this feeling and resistance a necessary concomitant of pastoral care? Perhaps it cannot be removed completely, but it can be reduced to a great extent. There are two reasons for this possibility. The first is the fact that care, including pastoral care, is something universally human. It is going on in every moment of human existence. The second more important reason is that care is essentially mutual; he who gives care also receives care. In most acts of taking care of someone, it is possible for the person who is the object of care to also become a subject.

Tillich suggests that without this mutuality we "fall into another form of objectification, which is the great curse of our industrial society." One result of this objectification is severe damage to a person's self-awareness, and, according to Tillich, is a problem that:

applies to all forms of taking care of someone, be it the social, the educational, the political, the medical, or the psychotherapeutic function. In all of them the heart of the subject-object problem is of decisive importance.

As I will further describe below in the review of McKnight's book, objectification is exactly what took place as the culture moved from an industrial to a service-based society. Service, often labeled "care," becomes a commodity. Sick neighbors become patients or clients. To the degree such occurs (and many argue that it is the *sine qua non* of modern health care), Christian, Jewish, and Muslim pastoral caregivers will be compromised! Those traditions insist on honoring the "person" as integral to all else.

Pastoral care givers will also be compromised in another significant way. Tillich further argued that: ". . . . A pastor engaged in pastoral care is a helper in a situation in which the relation to the ultimate has become a problem, and this problem is in every human being." In an issue of the journal titled *Christian Bioethics* reviewed below, the authors note that such a clear and strong theological foundation is foreign to many of today's chaplains. Instead, pastoral care has evolved into a "Generic Chaplaincy" that moves away from a cognitive-based approach that grapples with the I-Thou to a feeling-based one. In a response to Tillich's paper, James M. Gustafson labeled such feeling-based approaches as "pseudo-charismatic manipulation"! However, since many (if not most) of our theological concepts are understood noetically, this approach invites any whose "heart" is in the right place or who have a "calling" for it to deliver pastoral care. (Might this partially explain the present interest among nurses, social workers, and others to provide spiritual care?)

2. "How My Mind Has Changed Regarding Pastoral Care." Granger E. Westberg. *Lutheran Quarterly;* May, 1967 Volume XIX, Number 2.

One of the challenges Dr. Westberg identified is similar to that of Tillich, namely, "As ministers of God, how do we translate what they consider to be a secular problem into its theological dimensions to help them see that God is involved in all of life . . . ?" A second challenge concerned where education and training for such ministry should occur. Grateful to the hospitals and prisons that had opened their doors to clergy education programs, Westberg believed it should return to the parish. Many benefits would accrue from such a locus. "Normalcy" rather than "pathology" would be the context for the conversations. This might help recapture the notion of "spiritual direction" (which is an egalitarian relationship) rather than "pastoral counsel" (which easily becomes a power relationship of expert-client). And, religious language could return to the dialogue in the parish. Westberg was concerned that in clinical settings, "We modern ministers steer clear of cramming religion down people's throats. So we went to the other extreme and never even mentioned religion."

Westberg closed his article with a quote from British theologian Frederic Greeves (*Theology and the Cure of Souls.* London, Epworth Press, 1960) that is equally relevant today. Greeves mentions that many in mental health welcomed ministerial assistance even though they do not accept the beliefs that are foundational to that assistance. He then asks:

> Is this a point of view which we, as Christians, ought to tolerate and encourage, however flattering it may be to think that we are wanted? Is not a use of religion as a way to mental health, in spite of the fact that religious beliefs are judged to be purely "mythological" (in the sense of being untrue), a way of reducing Christianity to magic, a way which we should have to repudiate even if we were persuaded that it would produce beneficial results? The way back to a specifically pastoral ministry is a long one. . . . But would not this subterfuge be but a new version of other ways of inviting men to God under false pretenses, a modern counterpart of the meal plus evangelism, or the youth club with religion carefully concealed, [both] methods which have proved their worthlessness? Do we not make it harder rather than easier for men and women to see and find the health which is often very different from what many would call full physical and mental health, the health which God makes possible? Why do so many of us seem almost to be ashamed of being the kind of specialist that we are supposed to be?

3. John McKnight. *The Careless Society: Community and Its Counterfeits.* Basic Books, New York, 1996.

In the Introduction McKnight asks: "How is it that America has become so dispirited?" As evidence he lists the problems of families, growing violence, failing schools, medical systems out of control, and others. And, he suggests, "the most common response is a call for institutional reform. Leaders urge Total Quality Management programs, new technologies, 'right-sizing,' lifelong learning, and new highways for information that will renew the services produced by our systems." These reforms will all fail, according to McKnight. And, the reasons they will fail also suggest the path "that will allow us to create an effective, satisfying society." "Our problem," he says, "is weak communities, made ever more impotent by our strong service systems." Sounding Tillichian, he goes on:

> Service systems can never be reformed so they will "produce" care. Care is the consenting commitment of citizens to one another. Care cannot be produced, provided, managed, organized, administered, or commodified. Care is the only thing a system cannot produce. Every institutional effort to replace the real thing is a counterfeit? Care is, indeed, the manifestation of a community.

The four "counterfeiting aspects" of society that contribute to our modern dilemma have direct ties to modern professional chaplaincy/ pastoral care: professionalism, medicine, human service systems, and the criminal justice system. Each of these is discussed in depth, both as to the usual benign way they began and the terrible consequences they can generate.

Professionalism is certainly a subject that is dear to pastoral care. Considerable individual and organizational energies have been directed towards the establishment of a pastoral care that is "professional!" Yet, many suggest that such a development or establishment leads to the iatrogenic problems almost always generated in power relationships. While such power abuses are not new, they are made more dangerous due to the major changes in 20th century Western culture. At the beginning of this century, 90% of the work force was in manufacturing and 10% in services. On the eve of the 21st century those proportions are reversed! This has considerable political and economic significance. We need to keep a healthy professionalism to keep the economy going. So, there is a dependence "upon the manufacture of need and the definition of new deficiencies." This is not to paint a diabolical face on the professional. As McKnight suggests in his Chapter, "Professionalized Services and Disabling Help," it is a natural consequence when service becomes business, clients become consumers, and persons are hired to market services. And, to "mask" the economic factors involved, we call it "care." That word, per McKnight, is a "potent political symbol." What is not so clear is that its use masks the political interests of servicers. This fact is further obscured by the symbolic link between care and love. The result is that the politico-economic issues of service are hidden behind the mask of love. Behind that mask is simply the servicer, his systems, techniques, and technologies–a business in need of markets, professionals in need of an income.

It is crucial that we understand that this mask of service is not a false face. The power of the ideology of service is demonstrated by the fact that most servicers cannot distinguish the mask from their own face. Thus, to be successful as a professional, one must convince one's "customers" that there is a "need"–and that "need" can best, if not only, be serviced by the professional. And, those needs and services must be measurable, quantifiable. This suggests to this reviewer why many of the "reforms" in modern healthcare so often impact chaplains and pastoral care. Post-modern religion suggests that, at most, our need vis-à-vis God is to accept that S/He loves us as the default position and that nothing that is happening to us has any connection to that relationship. So, we need a cheerleader form of pastoral care, one who keeps us from sinking into any Jobian or Pauline thinking!

The chapters on "Medicine," "Human Service Systems" and the "Criminal Justice Systems" paint a similarly challenging picture. Perhaps at no other time in human history have the "servicers" been such a dominant factor and so the challenges are new. The concluding Chapter, "On the Backwardness of Prophets," is one which speaks directly to the truths of our religious heritages as Christians (I need to hear if it speaks to my Jewish and Muslim brothers/sisters as well). He sees this in Christ's imperative to be servants, not lords. Thus, as Christians we might celebrate the growth of service in this century, but also be fully aware of its problems. After all, there are good servants and bad servants. McKnight: "I wonder whether the human reality is always to make servanthood into lordship. It may be that there is no way to define service so that we will not get it backwards and make it a system of control" (That sounds close to the concept of original sin!). McKnight believes that such may be the reason why Jesus, in the final instructions to the disciples, says: "No longer do I call you servants. . . . I call you friends . . . " (John 15.15).

Perhaps beyond the revolution of Christian service is the final revolution, the possibility of being friends. Friends are people who know, care, respect, struggle, love justice, and have a commitment to each other through time. Friends are people who understand that it is not servants–the professors, lawyers, doctors, and teachers–who make God's world. Rather, friends are people who understand that it is through their mutual action that they become Christians. Christ's mandate to be friends is a revolutionary idea in our serving society. . . . Why friends rather than servants? Perhaps it is because He knew that servants could always become lords but that friends could not. Servants know the mysteries that can control those to whom they give help. Friends are people who know each other. They are free to give and receive help. In our time, professionalized servants are people who are limited by the unknowing friendlessness of their help. Friends, on the other hand, are people liberated by the possibilities of knowing how to help each other.

4. H. Tristram Engelhardt (Ed.). "Generic Chaplaincy: Providing Spiritual Care in a Post-Christian Age" *Christian Bioethics: Non-Ecumenical Studies in Medical Morality.* 1998, Volume 4(3).

Engelhardt begins this provocative journal issue with these words: "Religion-non-specific, denominationally neutral hospital chaplaincy, a generic chaplaincy, has been integrated into the health care services of many hospitals. It provides spiritual care without religious specificity to members of whatever denominations are encountered."
The genesis of such a development is linked to the:

> professional setting in which chaplains find themselves in many American hospitals. They have been hired to provide spiritual care, but the nature of that care is left strategically under-defined . . . . Ministers who were once ordained in particular religions are reprofessionalized into trans-denominational roles. Institutional expectations reshape their vocation into the role of generic chaplains.

This development has made it easier for chaplains to take a stance on a par with colleagues in the health care fields.

> Their services are part of the health care team. They are not the services of a person on a divine mission sent into the hospital to

bring salvation. . . . Such a view . . . involves a foundational shift in the understanding of the role and significance of spiritual ministry. The focus of the chaplain is no longer on providing care from the richness of a particular religion, but rather on transcending religious or denominational boundaries to reach out to anyone in spiritual need.

Few in any of the professional chaplain organizations would proudly accept themselves as "generic." Denominational endorsement suggests, at the very least, that specificity has some role to play. Certification processes also engage the chaplain in some theological process so as to determine whether s/he has some foundational assumptions about God, life, healing, etc.

Yet, it may be possible that the endorsement-certification exercise exists parallel to the day-to-day practices and functions. Possible? Probable? It is increasingly probable at least in many of the healthcare facilities as staff struggle with personnel shortages, extremely short patient stays, greater utilization of out-patient or ambulatory services, less active involvement with community clergy, etc. Wrestling with ultimate questions (à la Tillich) does not lend itself to drive-thru pastoral care!

This journal issue concerning generic chaplaincy arose out of an actual case "of conflict over the authority, usefulness, and place of generic chaplaincy" and it could be the focus for an entire unit of Clinical Pastoral Education or a series of discussions with parish clergy. Only two chapters are mentioned here because they speak to issues raised in these reviews.

In "A Christian for the Christians, a Muslim for the Muslims?" Kurt W. Schmidt and Gisela Egler address the problem of "absolutism"–i.e., the claim that Christ is essential for salvation. "Various models have been proposed to help Protestant chaplains find an authentic form of pastoral care suitable for all religions. Until a clear position is assumed with regard to Christianity's demand of absolutism, however, none of these approaches can be satisfactory."

In multi-cultural societies, today's politically correct, economically challenged and litigative-sensitive healthcare facility does exert a pressure on pastoral care persons to "please" all customers. Rarely is that pressure overt. If it were, at least the chaplain's challenge would be clearly defined. Rather the pressures are subtle and masked. Budgets can be cut rather than facing issues directly. Then, when hiring freezes thaw, new chaplains can be employed who are more open to bringing generic warmth, support, and care to the patients.

In another chapter, Joseph J. Kotva, Jr. suggests a model for chaplaincy called "Agapeic Intervention." He begins with an excellent overview of the reasons why Generic Chaplaincy has arisen, as well as the dangers. Yet, he believes the need for chaplaincy is so great that the risks must be faced. To minimize the dangers, he offers an approach modeled after the Mennonite's vocation of service to the poor and suffering. The intention of "Agapeic Intervention" is to be "catalytic and dialogical" rather than respectful and sympathetic. Such would require chaplains to have clear self-identities, be willing to sincerely identify with the "other," and be willing to share frankly and intelligently. They would not seek the lowest common denominator. The problem is whether such a chaplain could be a hired or even serve in today's hospital. He agrees, and suggests that perhaps "we need to rethink how chaplains are paid and placed. Such rethinking would encourage a non-generic chaplaincy."

In summary, the materials reviewed above raise some of the questions that must be faced if professional chaplaincy is to continue into the 21st century. Perhaps some chaplains will answer that they will not face these questions. However, if we chose to struggle we will bring healing to ourselves–and at least serve as a hope to the many physicians, nurses and other healthcare colleagues who similarly struggle in the institutions who treat the sick.

Frank S. Moyer, MDiv, BCC
Professional Pastoral Resources
Rockford, IL
PadreEthic@aol.com

CURRENT CONTENTS IN THE LITERATURE CONCERNING HEALTH CARE REFORM OF IMPORTANCE TO PROFESSIONAL CHAPLAINS

Introduction

W. Noel Brown, STM, BCC, Editor

Since the early 1990s, downsizing (or "rightsizing," the euphemisms for layoffs being plentiful) has been common in the health care sector. However, there has been surprisingly little written about it by chaplains. This work represents the first effort to gather in one place some reflections and resources for those who are affected by these changes and wish to plan a strategic response.

It is no mystery why so little has been written. Whether the change came relentlessly, inevitably and was foreseen months before the cuts were made, or if the cuts were totally unexpected, the effects on the persons involved are the same. For those downsized, there is depression and anger and anxiety. For those who retain their positions, parallel feelings often arise as they wonder "will I be next?" Neither group

W. Noel Brown is affiliated with Pastoral Services & Education, Northwestern Memorial Hospital, Feinberg 16-706, 251 Huron Street, Chicago, IL 60611.

[Haworth co-indexing entry note]: "Current Contents in the Literature Concerning Health Care Reform of Importance to Professional Chaplains." Brown, W. Noel. Co-published simultaneously in *Journal of Health Care Chaplaincy* (The Haworth Pastoral Press, an imprint of The Haworth Press, Inc.) Vol. 10, No. 1, 2000, pp. 79-84; and: *Professional Chaplaincy: What Is Happening to It During Health Care Reform?* (ed: Larry VandeCreek) The Haworth Pastoral Press, an imprint of The Haworth Press, Inc., 2000, pp. 79-84. Single or multiple copies of this article are available for a fee from The Haworth Document Delivery Service [1-800-342-9678, 9:00 a.m. - 5:00 p.m. (EST). E-mail address: getinfo@haworthpressinc.com].

seems interested in actually writing about the subject. I know this from personal experience because I was downsized out of my position in the summer of 1999.

A computerized search of the pastoral care literature in The Orere Source and Medline revealed a small number of articles from the past decade. Setting aside those that were related to aspects of managed care as it affects doctors and their practice of medicine, and also the ethical issues of managed care, the literature can usefully be separated into four general categories.

1. The Effects of Downsizing

At one level, the effects of downsizing are obvious if one focuses on the psychological effects of those affected both directly and indirectly. It is largely negative (Moore et al. 1996; Vahtera et al. 1997; Petterson & Arnetz 1998; Corey-Lisle et al. 1999). It is within these articles that chaplains will find descriptions of the impact of downsizing.

Within the last two years, as the cuts in the numbers of health care providers have deepened, authors seek to better understand a number of unknowns, such as the relationships between staff numbers and patient safety, whether retraining staff for multiple tasks is always beneficial, whether the marketing model can be applied to health-care delivery in a pure form, and whether there have been significant financial gains as a result of downsizing anyway (Gable-Rodriguez 1993; Bellandi 1998; Heimoff 1998; Woodard et al. 1998; Anonymous 1998 & 1999; Brownell et al. 1999; Woodward et al. 1999). These articles are included to broaden the chaplain's perspective on downsizing, including the many unanswered questions.

2. What Is Lost When Chaplaincy Departments Are Downsized?

The answer to this question may again seem self-evident, linked as it is to the very raison d'être of chaplaincy. But chaplains must remember that we live and function in an era where there is "a Pharaoh who knows not Joseph." Because of the wholesale re-examining of health care delivery from efficiency and economic perspectives, as well as the on-going revolution in the technical delivery of medical therapeutic power, pastoral care is being scrutinized as never before. In order to withstand such review, the chaplaincy profession must be able to examine itself and interpret the findings about its own practices to administrators who may wish to label pastoral care as ephemeral.

What does chaplaincy contribute to the bottom line–and how? In some settings, institutions gather information about patient satisfaction and these results can be helpful. However, it appears that it is mainly in not-for-profit institutions where the hospital is closely tied to the community that this information is being gathered.

Patients are generally very favorably disposed towards chaplains and their ministry (Gibbons et al. 1991). Administrators, too, are generally positive toward the work of their chaplains (Manns 1990). This will, however, not necessarily ensure that when choices must be made they will leave a department adequately staffed to provide an effective ministry, or even leave a department at all. The experience in Georgia's state facilities in the early 1990s teaches that lesson.

Higdon (1994) has described the effects of the downsizing in her institution. Derrickson and Derrickson (1994-5) have looked at the future to describe the options they see as possibilities for chaplaincy. Research will hopefully continue to be done that demonstrates the value of pastoral care either financially or in terms of what patients and their families value within the care they receive. We must also find a way of talking to hospital administrators, using language that will assist them to understand the nature of the "softer" contributions made by chaplains to patient care–the value of support, the power of love, caring, forgiveness, meaning-making, grief resolution, reconciliation (Jacques 1993; Jones & Alexander 1993; Wetzler 1994). These are all contributions made by the modern trained chaplain, and they are all activities that are lost when a pastoral care department is downsized. But it is only in the last years of this century that our own intuitive knowledge of the importance of these contributions has been supported by the scientific research that has now been done concerning each of them. (See Note 1.)

3. Ministry in the Institution to Those Still Employed

There appears to be only two articles written by chaplains about ministry to staff and the organization as a community after a reduction in numbers (Tripp 1990; Driscoll 1998). There is, however, some useful material describing activities directed at either individuals, groups and the institution as a whole that has been written by other health care professionals (Vogelsang 1992; Godfrey 1994; Tyrrell 1994; Hauser 1996; Veninga 1997; Bumbaugh 1998; Rondeau 1998).

The insights of this group of authors will need to be transformed into the culture and style of the individual chaplain, depending upon their place and roles within their own organization, not to mention their own proclivity to providing pastoral care away from the bedside.

4. Ministry to the Administration of the Institution

There is little written from a theological perspective concerning the role of administrators. One notable exception is an interview by Joseph Driscoll with a Chicago hospital CEO (1995). Also a paper by Quick et al. (1992) sketches some themes that will alert chaplains to areas of pastoral care with administrative teams.

END THOUGHTS

There are no "sacred cows" left in health care systems, a truth that should have become self-evident to chaplains after the downsizing in Georgia in August 1991. If downsizing can take place in the "Bible-belt" and so thoroughly, it can happen anywhere. But this reality does not relieve chaplains of the tasks of interpreting their work and its value in terms that will make sense to administrators. Some valuable work has already been done by VandeCreek, Fitchett, Burton, Berg and others. The task now consists of finding ways to share the burden of interpreting our ministry across the profession with every chaplain taking what has already been discovered about best practices in pastoral care, and finding ways of both enacting, and interpreting those actions in their own situation. And if a chaplain cannot do that, there is advice from Garrison Keillor; see the title of the reference (1996).

NOTES

1. The Orere Source can be contacted at <oreresource@rocketmail.com>. The web-site for Medline is at <http://www.ncbi.nlm.nih.gov/PubMed/>.

2. Not included in this overview is any reference to the work that has been done by chaplains themselves to substantiate the value of chaplaincy to individual patients and family members. There is a growing body of research on this subject which can be located with the help of pastoral care databases containing references to this information. See either Medline or The Orere Source.

REFERENCES

Anonymous, 1998. Reengineering survey finds changes vary widely, as do resulting financial benefits. *Health Care Cost Reengineering Reports* 3(11) 171-3.

Anonymous, 1999. New marketing strategy has CA hospital saying 'in with the old and out with the new.' *Health Care Cost Reengineering Reports* 4(3) 43-7.

Bellandi, D. 1998. The quiet restructuring. Blaming feds, hospitals shed workers, facilities in droves, *Modern Healthcare* 28(50) 2-3, 16.

Brownell, M.D., Roos, N.P., & Burchill, C. 1999. Monitoring the impact of hospital downsizing on access to care and quality of care. *Medical Care* 37(6Suppl) JS135-150.

Bumbaugh, M. 1998. Moving beyond survival after downsizing. *Nursing Management* 29(2) 30-33.

Corey-Lisle, P. & Tarzian, A.J. et al. 1999. Healthcare reform. Its effects on nurses. *J. of Nursing Administration*, 29(3) 30-7.

Derrickson, B. & Derrickson, P. 1994-5. Assessing pastoral care services for the future. *CareGiver Journal* 11(1) 26-32.

Driscoll, J.J. 1995. Truth-telling: CEO ties truth-telling to respect for partners. *Vision* 5(6) 5-8.

Driscoll, J.J. 1998. Worries in the workplace. *Vision* 8(7) 4-5.

Gable-Rodrigues, J. 1993. Shifting paradigms–Care 2000: A chaplain's perspective. *J. of Pastoral Care* 47(4) 421-424.

Gibbons, J.L., Thomas, J., VandeCreek, L. & Jesson Arne K. 1991. The value of hospital chaplains: patient perspectives. *J. of Pastoral Care* 45(2) 117-126.

Godfrey, C. 1994. Downsizing: coping with personal pain. *Nursing Management* 25(10) 90-93.

Hauser, L. 1996. Reigning the spirit in the work place. *The 1996 University Associates Annual: Training* 26(1) 297-303.

Heminoff, S. 1998. Voices from the front-line. 14-hospital study concludes the results of reengineering have been "very, very mixed." *Strategic Healthcare Excellence* 11(10) 1-6.

Higden, T. 1994. The impact of a cost effectiveness program on pastoral services: one department's experience. *CareGiver Journal* 11(1/2) 27-37.

Jacques, R. 1993. Untheorized dimensions of caring work: caring as a structural practice and caring as a way of seeing. *Nursing Administration Quarterly* 17(2) 1-10.

Jones, C.B., & Alexander J.W. 1993. The technology of caring: a synthesis of technology and caring for nursing administration. *Nursing Administration Quarterly* 17(2) 11-20.

Keillor, G. 1996. You say potato. . . . and I say leave the downsized life behind and head for where the caribou roam. *The Family Therapy Networker* 20(5) 17.

Manns, M., 1990. The valuation of pastoral care by hospital administrators: a survey of selected for-profit and not-for-profit institutions. *J. of Health Care Chaplaincy* 3(1) 5-22.

Moore, S., Kuhrik, M., & Katz, B. 1996. Coping with downsizing. *Nursing Management* 27(3) 28-29.

Petterson, I.L., & Arnet, B.B. 1998. Psychosocial stressors and well-being in health care workers. The impact of an intervention program. *Society, Science, and Medicine* 47(11) 1763-1772.

Quick, D.L., Nelson, D.L., Joplin, J.R., & Quick, J.D. 1992. Emotional isolation and loneliness: executive problems. *The 1992 University Associates Annual: Developing Human Resources* 21, 165-174.

Rondeau, K. 1998. Treating victims and survivors with respect when downsizing is necessary. *Healthcare Management Forum* 11(4) 6-11.

Tripp, K.F. 1990. Ministry in a climate of grief. *Health Progress* 71(2) 74-76.

Tyrrell, R.A. 1994. Life after downsizing: strategies for organizational healing and revitalization. *Medsurgical Nursing* 3(5) 363-366.

Vahtera, J., Kivimaki, M., & Pentti, J. 1997. Effect of organizational downsizing on health of employees. *The Lancet* 350(9085) 1124-1128.

Veninga, R.L. 1997. After the downsizing. *Health Progress* 78(5) 14-17, 20.

Vogelsang, J.D. 1992. Healing the organization: reconstruction in times of crisis. *J. of Religion and Health* 31(4) 343-351.

Wetzler, H.P. 1994. A way to measure value. *Healthcare Forum Journal* 37(4) 45-49.

Woodward, B., Fottler, M.D., & Kilpatrick, A.O. 1998. Transformation of an academic medical center: lessons learned from restructuring and downsizing. *Health Care Management Review* 24(1) 81-94.

Woodward, C.A., & Shannon, H.S. et al. 1999. The impact of re-engineering and other cost reduction strategies on the staff of a large teaching hospital: a longitudinal study. *Medical Care* 37(6) 556-569.

Index

Australian chaplaincy
  utility research, 40ff
  downsizing of, 43ff
    and religious volunteers, 42ff

Chaplaincy, generic, 75-77
Chaplaincy funding, 53-67
  variations in, 53ff

Downsized: *See also* Health Care
    Reform
Downsizing of chaplaincy departments
  admonishing peer directors, 32ff
  anger about, 4
  department characteristics and, 12ff
  importance of department visibility,
    24ff
  in Australia, 43ff
  institutional characteristics and,
    12ff
  ministry to hospital staff, 33ff
  need for administrative support,
    21ff
  need to embrace change, 27ff
  personal experience of, 1ff

  personal learning from, 5ff
  public response to, 4
  related to department size, 10ff
  related to CPE programs, 12ff
  strategies to defend against, 13ff
  threats in the future, 13ff
Downsizing Committee, xiii

Economic rationalism, 37-52
  and value of hospital chaplaincy,
    39ff
  and hospital chaplincy funding, 42ff

Health Care Reform
  department director responses to,
    21-36
  impact on pastoral care
    departments, 7ff
  looking beyond the symptoms, 69-73
  other literature regarding, 79-84

Qualitative research, 19-36

Religious volunteers, 42ff